Tapping the Power of PowerPoint for Medical Posters and Presentations

Anand J. Thakur

Tapping the Power of PowerPoint for Medical Posters and Presentations

Springer

Anand J. Thakur
Department of Orthopedics
Polyclinic Irla
Mumbai, India

ISBN 978-981-19-1815-5 ISBN 978-981-19-1816-2 (eBook)
https://doi.org/10.1007/978-981-19-1816-2

This Springer imprint is published by the registered company Springer Nature Singapore Pte Ltd.
The registered company address is: 152 Beach Road, #21-01/04 Gateway East, Singapore 189721, Singapore

To
Dr Rajeshwar Singh
Medical writer
Friend and mentor

Preface

My interest in medical presentations dates back to my post-graduate training in orthopaedics in the late 1960s. Making a slide was an elaborate process: once the text for a slide was finalized, a medical artist prepared an art work. After the author had edited, artwork was photographed. Slides were classified as positive—black image on white background; negative—white image on black background; diazo-chrome white image on blue background; and true colour slides. Black and white slides were easiest to procure. Further processing with diazo dyes produced classic blue background and text appearing in white. The colour transparency films were expensive and were used for special lectures. All slides were mounted in a frame and placed sequentially in a special carrier box for projection. Upside down projections were common. The number of slides used was limited. In the early 1980s, I organized a symposium on medical slides with the help of my friend Rajeshwar Singh who owned a medical advertisement studio. In one of the talks, I declared, 'there are seven ways of projecting a slide wrongly and only one correct method'. Over the years, I accumulated considerable information on presentation skills and gave several seminars on the subject. Everything changed in the early 1990s with the advent of a personal computer. First to go was the medical artist because I could make artwork using a program 'Harvard Graphics' and convert it to a transparency for projection. This further changed with the availability of PowerPoint and digital projectors. It was now easy to churn out innumerable slides, comfortably and at no extra cost. With Internet boom, the number of medical meetings exploded so did my urge to write down all the available material in an organized format for easy access and readability. Internet offers unlimited data on this subject which is scattered and disorganized. Learning from Internet blogs and YouTube videos is like 6 blind men examining an elephant; my book presents a 3D model that gives a total experience. It concentrates only on the 'why' aspect of creating a presentation; on 'how' to manoeuvre a presentation on a computer, there are several books and videos that are hard to match; a presenter is advised to refer to these.

This text is not for beginners. This is targeted at people who know how to handle a presentation program and have used it to make a few presentations. The writing is helpful for those who want their work to stand out in the crowd where hundreds of other presenters arc vying for attention by making a podium or poster presentation.

Modern presentation programs are very easy to use for all those who have elementary knowledge of a computer program. It is a good thing that the learning curve is very shallow to achieve basic level proficiency. The final product of a presentation program is a string of slides which have text and graphic material on it. Arranging text and pictorial material in an attractive style is a task that needs training in typography, designing, and display techniques. In the days before a personal computer, this was done by artists and printing professionals who had studied these disciplines and were well versed in proper ways of graphic display. These people had the equipment and knowledge to produce good pleasing layouts on paper. The computer has put the power of writing and display in the hands of people who do not have any training in typography, designing, and display. The result is a chaos; the audience has to tolerate badly displayed text and illustrations on the conference screen. Most such presentations have an amateurish look and are dull, even outright boring. A novice tends to use the templates provided with the program. These are unsuitable for medical presentations because they were created for presentation needs of the business world and are inadequate for healthcare presentations.

This text is a guide for people who want to make a presentation that audience will remember for some time. Following these simple rules and suggestions, the reader will be able to transform his mundane presentation to a magnificent one and be able to present his research with a flourish and make each of his presentation an unforgettable one.

I am thankful to Dr Narendra Agarwal of Springer Nature to accept my book proposal. Several of my friends made constructive suggestions for this project. I am grateful to Dilip Tanna, Kirit Vora, Nicholas Antao, Vikas Agashe, Neeraj Bijlani, Mahesh Kharde, Ashok Shyam, and Peter Anand for their friendly criticisms. Ravindra Pagare is my class mate from the early 1960s in medical college at Indore. After finishing as a Professor of ENT surgery, he has honed his creative skills and has become an accomplished cartoonist. He has drawn a few for the book which are delightful mood changers for the readers; I am grateful for his generosity. Another friend from the same era, Kirit Vora has been helping me in all my publications with his photo-editing skills and has done that again—thank you Kirit. The book was written during Covid lockdown. Though under considerable distress due to curbs on outdoor movements, my wife Urmila was considerate enough to allow me to pursue writing while she kept herself busy with TV serials and FaceTime. Apart from the cartoons, all the art work is mine, thanks to the digital era.

Mumbai, India Anand J. Thakur

Acknowledgement

Several of my friends, acquaintances, and fellow specialist have extended help in permitting me to use their photographs and slides for this work. I am listing their names in alphabetical order and specifying their contribution for copyright clarity.

Agashe VM Figs. 5.1, 9.8, 14.4, 14.6 and 14.7; Agashe Prachi Fig. 9.2f; Antao N Fig. 9.4; Bombay Orthopaedic Society Figs. 14.15 and 14.16; Damle Ajit Fig. 7.6; Jethwa J Figs. 10.3a and 10.7b; Makhecha M Fig. 9.6; Narvekar A D Fig. 9.2d; Pagare RN Figs. 1.2, 13.9, 14.8, 14.10, 14.1 and 14.14; Puri Ajay Video 7.2; Shah Siddharth Fig. 9.2a, b.

Contents

About the Author

Dr. Anand Thakur is currently in private practice in Mumbai and teaches postgraduate courses in orthopaedics. He received his MS ortho degree from the University of Bombay in 1970 and his MBBS degree from Mahatma Gandhi Memorial Medical College, Indore, in 1965. He has worked as a consultant orthopaedic surgeon at Cambridge Military Hospital, Aldershot, UK, and RN Cooper Municipal General Hospital, Juhu, Mumbai; he was a professor of orthopaedic surgery at GS Medical College, Parel, and the University of Bombay, Mumbai. He has authored three bestsellers, namely *Locking Plates: Concepts and Applications (2E)*, *Strategic Radiographic Positioning for Orthopedicians and Radiologists*, and *The Elements of Fracture Fixation (5E)*. He has also published several research papers in indexed journals.

Philosophy of Inception: Why a Book on Presentations

1

You are judged on the work you present, not the work you do; always take time to deliver high quality slides — Anonymous.

Contents

Despite a great proliferation of new media and technologies, the traditional live lecture is still highly regarded among medical professionals as an effective means of teaching and communication and the 'lantern slide' remains the most popular lecturer's aid. Today's healthcare professional in general, finds it almost impossible to communicate unless the lights are dimmed and there is picture on the screen. And not all of them do this competently (Fig. 1.1); some have developed this to a point where their presentation is little more than a slide show with an accompanying intangible narration

Fig. 1.1 Inept use of slides in a presentation

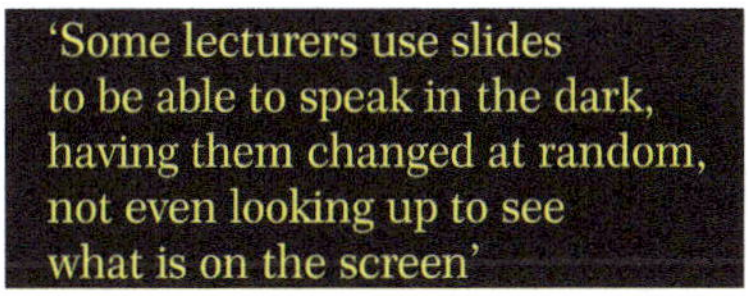

Supplementary Information The online version contains supplementary material available at [https://doi.org/10.1007/978-981-19-1816-2_1].

A. J. Thakur, *Tapping the Power of PowerPoint for Medical Posters and Presentations*, https://doi.org/10.1007/978-981-19-1816-2_1

Ascent of PowerPoint

A presentation software also known as program or App is a specialized software to create a slide show. It facilitates 3 things: (1) it allows addition and formatting of text, (2) there is method for entering and modifying graphic images, and (3) a slide show system to display the material. A slide show is a presentation of a prearranged sequence of still and video images on a screen. Slide shows originated in the 1600s as Magic Lantern slides and evolved from hand painted slides to photographic films mounted on glass, cardboard, and plastic slides. Its high point in the 1980s was slide boxes and carrousels mounted on highly luminous projectors. With the advent of computer technology slide making became easy and there was an explosion of slide presentations in every field of life and notably in science, medicine, finance and even in defence forces.

A computer slide show allows a presenter to match visual images to an oral presentation. A single image saves a presenter a thousand words of description. The flip side is the presenters show pictures and also speak thousands of words. When meticulously planned and executed, a presentation program is a powerful tool in the hands of medical speakers.

Presentation programs like Apple Keynote, Google Presentations, Prezi in general and PowerPoint in particular are user friendly apps. This is a good thing and this is a bad thing. Anyone with basic knowledge of the computer and keyboard can make a presentation using any of these programs in less than an hour. It is estimated that 300 million people use PowerPoint and 30 million presentations are created daily. A vast number of these presentations have template based slides with ornate backgrounds; the slides are text heavy and for emphasis presented in several typefaces and in multiple colours; display a long succession of baffling graphics that pixillate on projection; these were mostly downloaded from the web; the presenter simply using the text slides as teleprompter; use of several animation sequences merely to show prowess of the presentation app and serving no coherent purpose. Instead of using slides to punctuate and support the spoken word, too many of them are generated and into each too much information is stuffed. Eventually, the audience is left in a state of confusion and boredom as a sleep inducing presentation unfolds before a yawning audience; on occasions it could be worse—A Death by PowerPoint! Since 2001, this term is alluded to Angela R. Garber and is now used to describe any presentation that uses routine templates, dumps data, graphics, and text slides that tire even the most enthusiastic audience; a clear case of poor use of the presentation software (Fig. 1.2). For bad presentations PowerPoint or any other presentation program may not be blamed. Modern-day apps for presentation are of high intrinsic value and are products of hard and innovative work of hundreds of computer experts. For healthcare professionals use of presentation apps is a matter of survival and no longer a matter of choice.

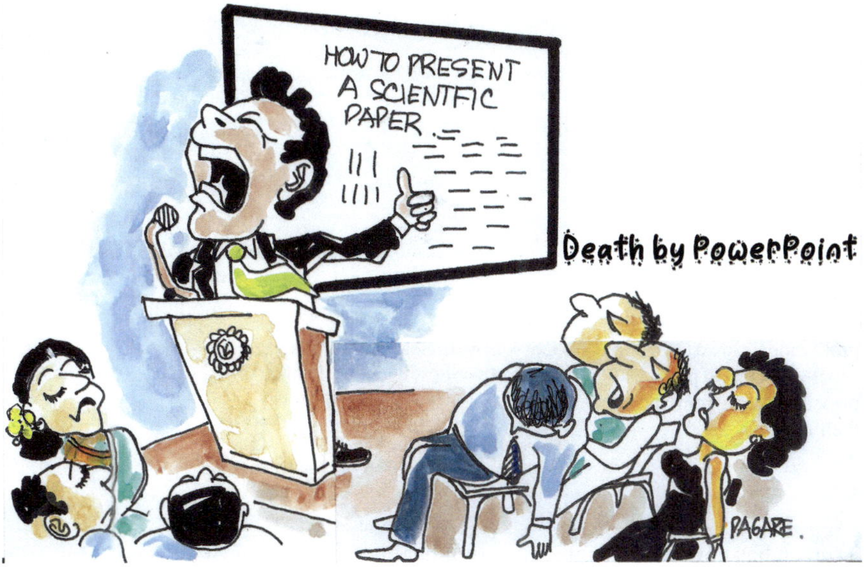

Fig. 1.2 'Death by PowerPoint'. A phrase expressing feelings of a jaded audience facing poorly made presentation in a boring lecture

History of PowerPoint

PowerPoint is a brainchild of Robert Gaskins. He as a computer scientist was perusing his PhD at Berkley. He also had background in presentation equipment as his father sold them. In 1984, he left his academic pursuits and joined a startup. Later he teamed up with developers Thomas Rudkin and Dennis Austin to create a presentation software to replace the use of older visual-aid technology, such as pamphlets, handouts, chalkboards, flip charts, posters, slides, and overhead transparencies. In 1985, the new program was christened Presenter and later reset to PowerPoint. Apple made its first venture capital investment in this App. Initially PowerPoint was made for Apple and Microsoft. The first two editions of the program were used on Apple Macintosh. Later Apple dropped it to develop Keynote. In 1986, many companies used the app to make presentations. In 1987, Microsoft purchased the app and refined it. Microsoft distributed its first official version of PowerPoint in 1990. By 1993, PowerPoint was making $100 million in sales annually. Today over one billion computers worldwide run PowerPoint (Fig. 1.3).

Audience information retention is superior when they simultaneously hear and see an object, educationists confirm. Healthcare professionals are lucky to be allowed to use presentation programs in their work (Fig. 1.4). Visual presentation on

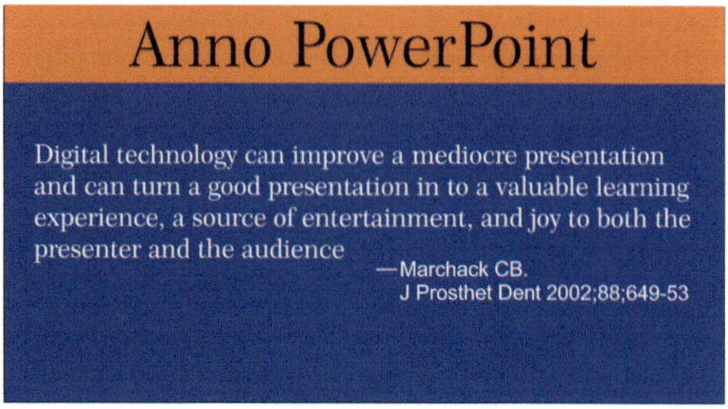

Fig. 1.3 Creation of PowerPoint had a lasting effect on the way people presented facts and data in a lecture

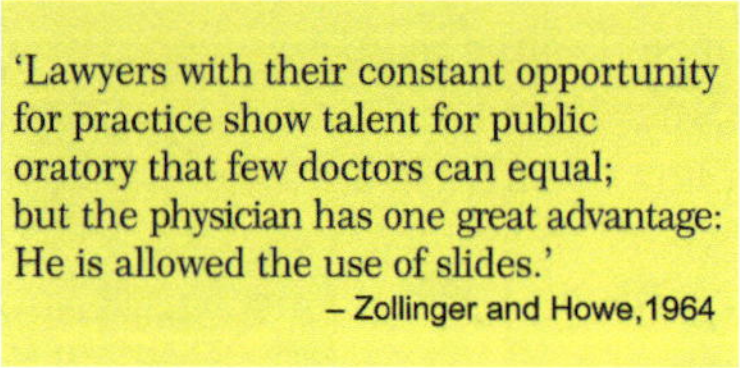

Fig. 1.4 Healthcare professionals are a privileged club to use a presentation program in their lectures

a screen has now become integral part of healthcare meetings of all genre. However, not all use it well. Some believe that simply displaying their ideas on screen will improve quality of their presentation. Usage of the presentation app is purposeful when it is used to put the subject in perspective, to distill evidence and to illustrate the results. Slides should complement a talk to give a truthful, exact, apt, and striking description of the matter being presented.

Why Does One Need Slides?

As a rule one use slides to reinforce and to supplement what one is saying; as a visual memory peg, to convey information rapidly, to save time in drawing, and to show examples or concepts that are difficult to describe in words (Fig. 1.5).

One should avoid use of slides as a prompt card; as a showcase for professional or personal travels; to show pictures of one's chance meeting with famous personalities; or use as fillers to flaunt one's collection of flowers because such display reduces the value and crispness of a presentation (Fig. 1.6). Filler slides work as diversion and do not help the presentation or hold audience attention (Video 1.1).

Essentials of a Good Slide

What makes a good slide? A slide should be appropriate for the subject being discussed; accurate for spelling and numbers; legible in choice of typeface, graphics; comprehensible in a short attention span; well executed in terms of technique; interesting enough to hold audience attention; and memorable for its aptness in the big picture (Video 1.2).

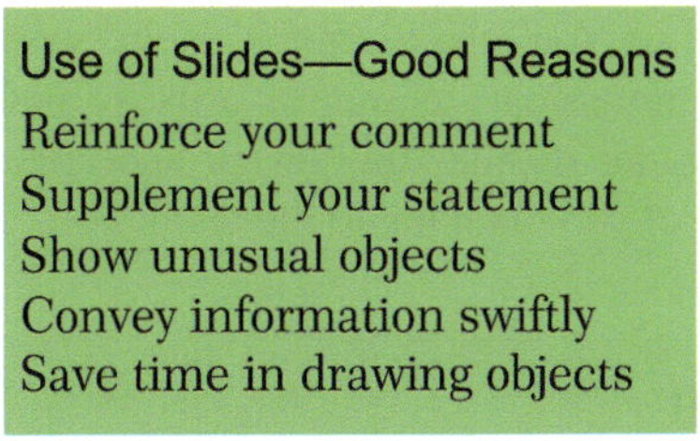

Fig. 1.5 Some agreeable instances to use slides in a lecture

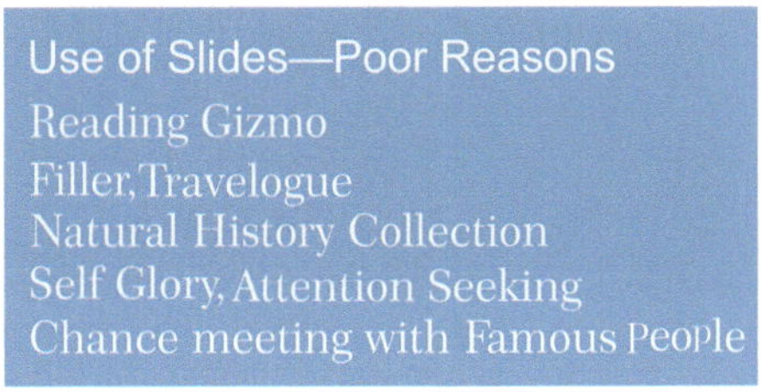

Fig. 1.6 A few awful circumstances to use slides in a lecture

Arranging text and pictorial material in an attractive style is a task that needs training in typography, designing, and display techniques. In the days before personal computer, this was done by artists and printing professionals who had studied these disciplines and were well versed in proper ways of graphic display. These people had the equipment and knowledge to produce good pleasing layouts on paper. The computer has put the power of writing and display in the hands of people who do not have any training in typography, designing, and display. It is essential to harness the power of a presentation program to one's benefit; to prepare a presentation that will be supportive to one's talk, keep the audience engaged, smoothly disperse one's ideas to the audience in an easy to assimilate form. Good medical presentations require long hours of hard work for meticulous planning, researching, fact-checking, and structuring.

What the Book Offers

In these writings I offer suggestions to help healthcare personnel and scientists to avoid common mistakes made in preparing and using computer-based presentations (Fig. 1.7). The book mainly deals with planning, design, and use of slides; more technical aspects of using a particular presentation know-how or a secret move are not the subject matter of this text because these are well dealt in easily accessible

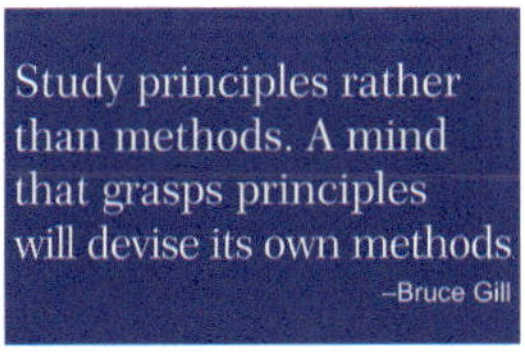

Fig. 1.7 Guiding principles of making presentations that engage audience attention in a conference are discussed in this book

bookstore literature, on YouTube, or in the 'Help' section of the program. Some of the readers may commission a computer artist to make the slides; however, it is essential that the reader dictates the design and contents leaving only the actual mechanical process of slide making to the techie.

Further Reading

Irwin T, Terberg J. Perfect medical presentations. Edinburgh: Churchill Livingstone Elsevier. 2004; isbn: 13:9780443074851

Optics of Slide Design & Projection

2

Contents

Resolution of Eyes

The sharpness of a projected digital image depends on how far away from the screen one is sitting, how good one's eyes are, and the native qualities of the image being projected on the screen.

How close two objects can become before they blur into one? At its best performance, human eyes can resolve two lines about 0.01 degrees apart: a 0.026 mm gap, 15 cm from one's face. More often, objects 0.04 mm wide (the width of a fine human hair) are just perceptible by good eyes, objects 0.02 mm wide are not. Generally speaking, human eye can recognize two lines, only when they subtend an angle of one degree or more (Fig. 2.1).

Optimum Viewing Comfort

In an auditorium an object can be seen comfortably when it reaches an angle within a range of 10–40 degrees at the eyes of the observer. An observer in the back row requires an angle of 10 degrees: so, the minimum height of a letter should be at least twenty percent of the screen. If the height of the picture is 2 metres, then the

A. J. Thakur, *Tapping the Power of PowerPoint for Medical Posters and Presentations*, https://doi.org/10.1007/978-981-19-1816-2_2

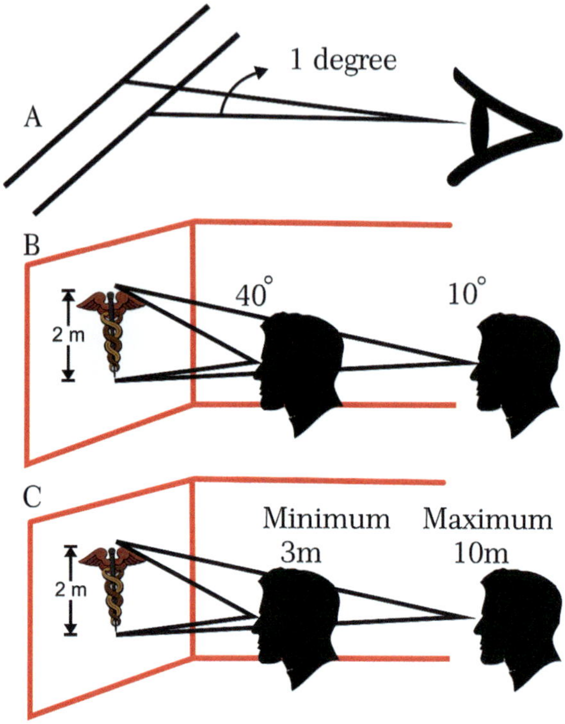

Fig. 2.1 (**a**) Objects must make an angle of 1 degree to be seen as separate items. (**b**) In an auditorium the figure on the screen is seen comfortably when it makes an angle between 40 and 10 degrees. (**c**) The range of comfortable viewing depends on the size of the image

minimum acceptable viewing distance is 3 metres and the longest viewing distance is only 10 metres. Any person sitting farther away will miss out on the details.

A different way of estimating the optimum audience viewing comfort from any screen is somewhere between two and six 'screen diagonals'. At a distance of less than two screen diagonals the images are likely to appear rough or out of focus. Beyond six diagonals, lettering will rapidly become too small to read (Fig. 2.2).

Not all seats in the above-described range offer undistorted view of the screen in the auditorium. Seats located within in a cone of 30° to 45° from the screen offer undistorted view. People sitting outside this funnel will have a suboptimal view of the screen. These guidelines help in establishing the necessary height and width of a viewing screen to project images which will subtend a comfortable viewing angle of 10° in the back rows of a conference hall.

Colour Vision Problems

8% of all adult males (females are carriers but 0.4% are affected) have colour vision problems. People with colour deficiencies generally do have some colour vision; they can tell differences between colours, but they do not see colours the same way as people with full colour vision (Fig. 2.3). Three types of colour vision deficiencies

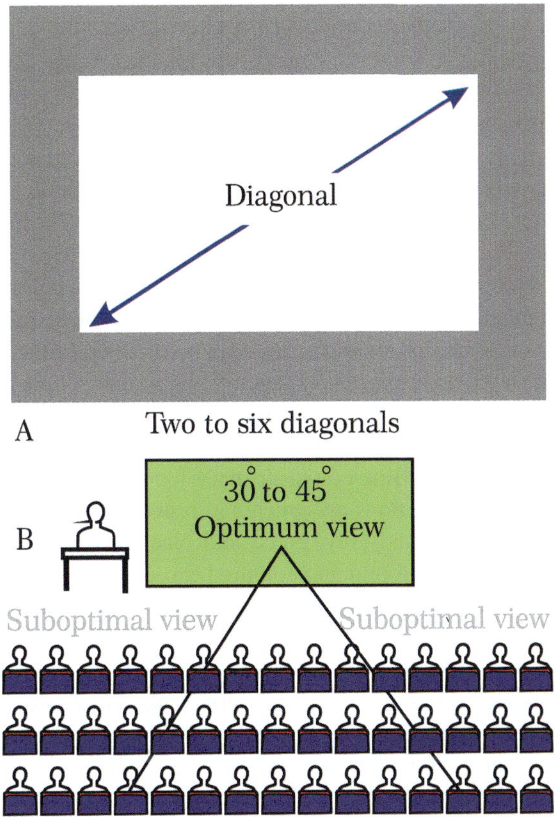

Fig. 2.2 Viewing is comfortable (**a**) when seated at a distance of two to six diagonals from the screen and (**b**) in a zone marked by 30 and 45 degree lines

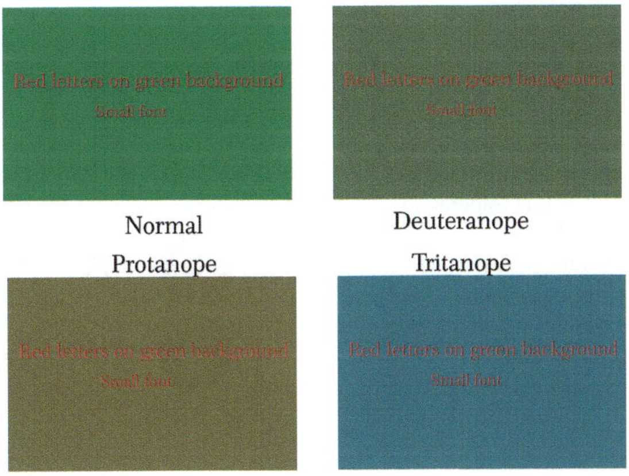

Fig. 2.3 A green and red graphic is seen differently by people suffering from 3 types of visual handicaps

are known: (1) Red and green colour deficit—Deuteranope, (2) A variant of red and green loss—Protanope, and (3) Uncommon blue and yellow colour deficiency—Tritanope. A normal vision person may not know what is a colour deficient view; Colour Blindness Simulator gives an authentic experience at http://www.color-blindness.com/coblis-color-blindness-simulator/. Whether a slide's contents are suitable for colour-blind audiences can be checked at this site: http://www.vischeck.com/vischeck/vischeckImage.php.; one needs to save a slide or entire presentation in png or jpeg format and upload it to vischeck. The answers are instantaneous. The site also provides means to make suitable changes to the colour combinations.

Inability to differentiate between some shades of green and of red is common in population at large. Using these colours to indicate positive and negative comments in a presentation should be avoided because a portion of audience may see the opposite of what is expected of them. To help such people the colour may be used with a text or an image, e.g. a green dot with text 'Yes' and tick sign (Fig. 2.4). Another common problem is the inability to tell blue shades from one another and from purple shades. Blue colour primary for text should be avoided. Other problematic colour combinations are green and brown, green and blue, blue and grey, blue and purple, green and grey, green and black, and light green and yellow. Generally, coloured background and coloured text cause legibility issues.

Dyslexic people have difficulty in accurate and fluent word recognition (Fig. 2.5). Dyslexia affects 1 in 10 adults to some degree; dyslexics find it difficult to read large blocks of text on a bright white screen. Short sentences with spacing of 1.5 or 2 is adequate for this class. Sans serif fonts suit dyslexics. Arial, Verdana, Tahoma, Century Gothic, and Trebuchet are well suited for them. Avoid condensed and cursive fonts, exception being Comic sans which is appreciated by this community. Underlining reduces readability by eliminating the recognition effect contributed by the descending elements of letters; underlining and italic fonts are difficult to read and so are the block capitals; bold lettering in sentence case is a good choice. These recommendations are good for dyslexic audience in particular and for others in general.

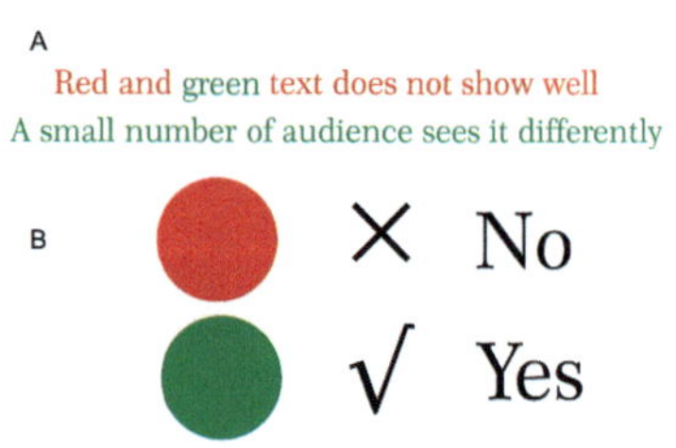

Fig. 2.4 (**a**) Red and green text is hard to read. (**b**) When it is imperative to use red and green colours for positive and negative comments, reiterate it with words and suggestive graphics

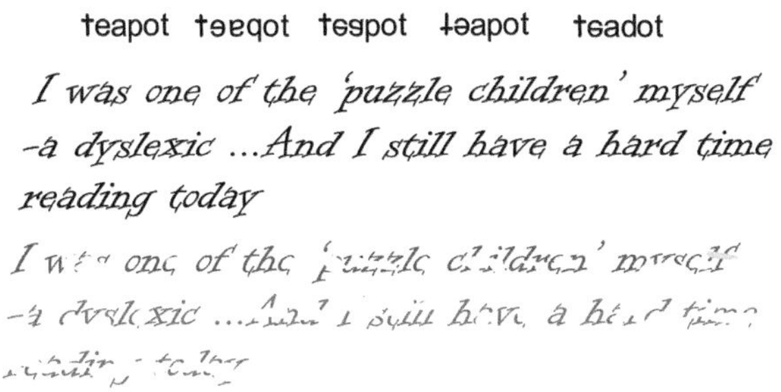

Fig. 2.5 Dyslexics see things differently

Pixel Explained

A digital image is formed by pixels—picture elements—Pictures shortened as pics; pix for picture was first used in 1932 in Variety magazine. Element shortened as el. The word Pixel was first used in 1965 in conjunction with digital imaging, then an emerging technology. IBM in 1972 used it for picture cell in their technical description of original PC. The term pixel is also used in other situations: printed pixels in a page, pixels on a display device, in a digital camera—six-megapixels—a nominal six million pixels, in an electronic signal, and as a unit of measure such as 20 pixels apart, 3200 pixels per inch or 480 pixels per line.

Pixel is the smallest unit of information in a digital image. A magnified image on a digital device breaks up into coloured squares—these are pixels (Fig. 2.6). Each pixel is made up of 3 sub-pixels, namely RGB (red, green, and blue); human eye cannot see these individual colours as they bled into a single tint at the pixel level.

An iPhone XI Pro has a pixel count of 2688 × 1242 and a resolution of 458 PPI. Pixel count is the image dimensions in pixels; horizontal pixels x vertical pixels. Resolution of the screen affects the appearance of an image; higher the resolution the sharper and crisper the image on the screen. These properties of a digital device are fixed and do not change. The pixel count of a digital image is modifiable and is controlled by the user. The picture size (also known as pixel count, resolution)—the physical number of pixels along the width and height—determines how the image looks on projection. More pixels per inch—PPI—allow for a continuous intermixture of colour and shape; the higher the PPI, the better the picture quality.

A disambiguation—the term Pixels Per square Inch (PPI) is used in two locations: to define the density of pixels within a digital image and the fixed number of pixels on a screen of a digital device. If an image with low pixel count and low PPI is projected on a large screen, the image is distorted or in technical terms, 'pixelation' occurs.

Once a larger image is scaled down and saved in a smaller size and lower resolution, considerable colour information is lost. Images for websites are saved at 72 PPI resolution. When such a small image is stretched for projection on a large 16:9 screen, its each colour pixel becomes larger to fill in the additional space causing image pixilation and distortion. One cannot expand a small, low-resolution image,

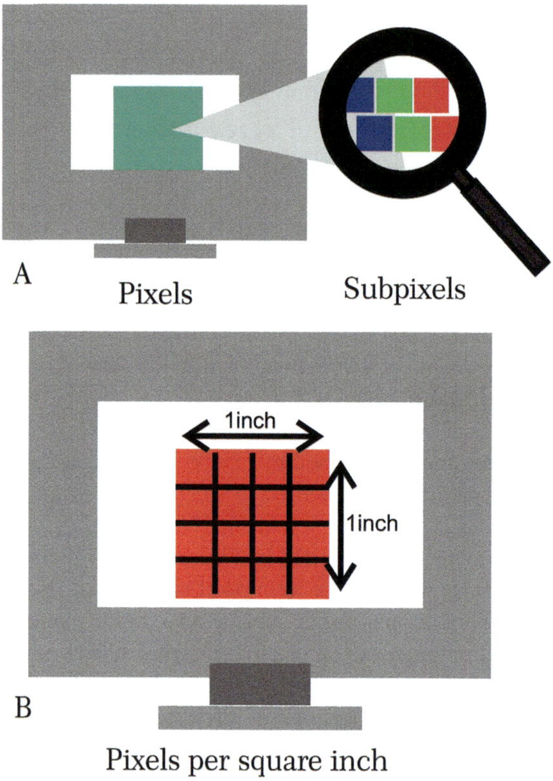

Fig. 2.6 (**a**) Pixel—Picture element—is the basic unit of a digital image (**b**) PPI—fixed number of pixels on a screen of a digital device

into a large stretched projected image and hope it appears as fine and as crisp as it was before it was down-scaled. It is now common to have conference screens in 16:9 ratio. For such screens, one should have an image with a pixel count of 1920 × 1080 and resolution of PPI 100 to 150. If one uses an image of 1028 × 768 to fit the same screen space, then pixilation is inevitable. Photo editing apps offer tools to change the image dimensions for presentation. 'Resampling' is ideal for decreasing the image dimensions for presentation. To expand a low-resolution image for projection 'resizing' utility should be used.

Resolution and Aspect Ratio

Resolution is a crucial word that applies to a computer and a digital projector (Fig. 2.7). Resolution is number of pixels, from side to side and top to bottom to create or project an image. More pixels mean a higher 'pixel density'and a crisper image. When the resolutions of the computer and the projector match, the image is crisp and fits the screen. 800 × 600, 1920 × 1080 (HD), 1920 × 1200, and 4 K × 2 K are popular resolutions. Second term associated with projection is aspect ratio. This

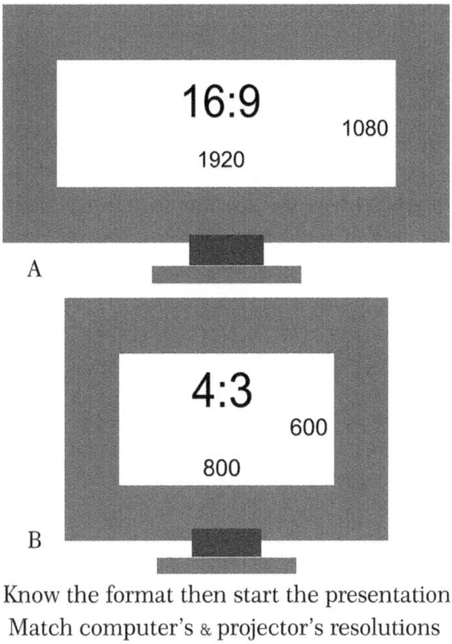

Fig. 2.7 (**a**) 16:9 wide screen slide size is presently extensively followed. (**b**) 4:3 standard slide size was popular in earlier generation of computers and projectors. Computer and projector resolutions should match for pleasing screen image

is the ratio between the image width and height; 4:3, 16:9, and 16:10 ratios are frequently used. An association exists between ratio and resolutions; 800 × 600 and 4:3 is a pair and so is 1920 × 1080 and 16:9; specifically, to create an image of 4:3 ratio, one requires 800 pixels horizontally and 600 pixels vertically. Higher resolution has more vertical and horizontal space on the screen; in lower resolutions items on the screen appear larger. When the projector resolution is lower than that of the computer, the image appears sharper on the computer's monitor than when projected on a screen.

It is wise to check in advance the projection parameters with conference organizers. One should prepare a presentation in the resolution and ratio given by the organizers, e.g. either 4:3 or 16:9. Changing the dimensions of the presentation afterwards is hard and may wreck a good slide design. Many times, the organizers are unable to tell beforehand the details of projection facilities. In that case one should opt for 16:9 ratio. It is easy to compress a slide without noticeable distortion. If a slide has to be enlarged from 4:3 to 16:9, then the computer has to double the pixels to fill the gap which it does in a complex way and may lead to significant distortions of graphics and text elements. Ultimate safe move is to prepare two sets of the presentation for different projection ratios.

If a presentation with videos and pictures has to be seen in a high-quality output, then it is necessary to set the slide ratio and computer resolutions similar to that of the projector. If there is a mismatch between the ratios and the resolutions of the computer and projector, then a presentation that looks great on the monitor will not look as good when projected on the screen.

Presentation Tenets

PNG and JPG formats are best suited for use in all presentation programs. These are light formats and do not increase the size of the presentation; TIFF files increase the size of the presentation and also slow down the slide show.

GIGO—Garbage in garbage out. When one puts much effort and time to prepare a presentation and puts one's prestige at stake, it is wise to use large, clear, and crisp images so the audience and presenter are pleased with the illustrations projected on the conference screens. Important presentation guidelines are illustrated in Fig. 2.8.

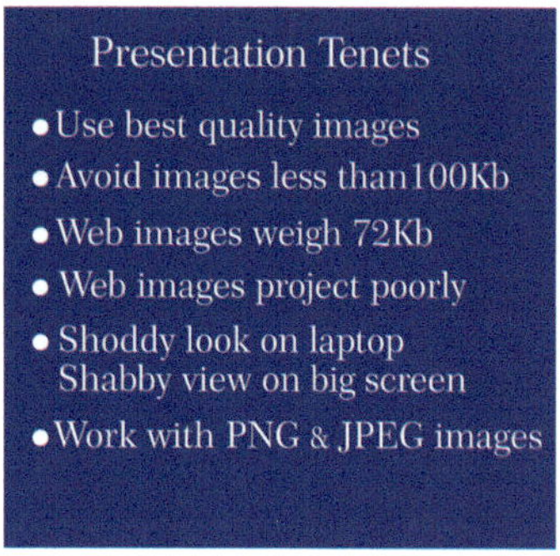

Fig. 2.8 A few principles of image selection for projection

Rational Use of Colour in Presentations 3

Why do two colours, put one next to the other, sing? Can one really explain this? No. – Pablo Picasso

Contents

Importance of Colour

Colour psychology rules high for marketing professionals but not so for healthcare personnel. However, choosing correct colours in the presentations enhances the effectiveness of the message and helps the audience in its comprehension.

People with diverse background take in colours differently. For example, red means robust to a healthcare provider, to an engineer it means hazard while a businessman perceives it as a loss-making item (Fig. 3.1).

There are 3 primary colours: red, blue, and yellow; these cannot be made by blending other colours. These three are basis for all other colours. Blending primary colours yields secondary colours: violet, orange, and green. Tertiary colours are created by combining a primary colour with secondary colours; outcome is six more colours, viz. red-orange, red-violet, blue-violet, blue-green, yellow-green, and yellow-orange. These 12 colours are represented in a colour wheel. In pure form a colour is known as hue. When white is mixed with a colour one gets a lighter colour known as tint. Mixing with grey creates a duller colour called tone. When black is added one gets a shade of that colour which is darker than the original. For convenience these colours are organized in a circle. Sir Isaac Newton first made this arrangement for the 7 spectrum colours; over the centuries, it has evolved to the present version (Fig. 3.2).

A. J. Thakur, *Tapping the Power of PowerPoint for Medical Posters and Presentations*, https://doi.org/10.1007/978-981-19-1816-2_3

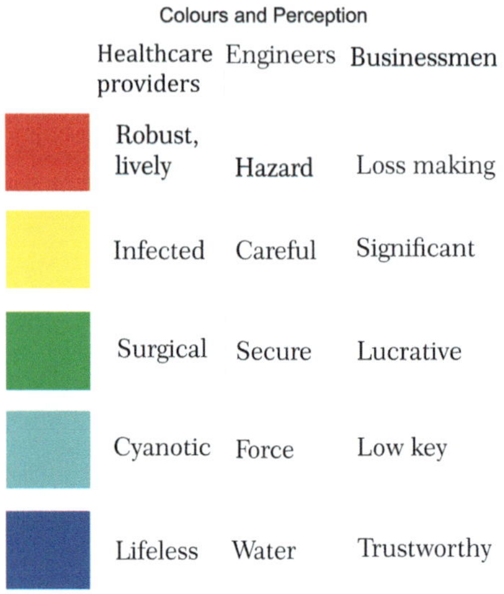

Fig. 3.1 Colour and its perception in people of varied callings

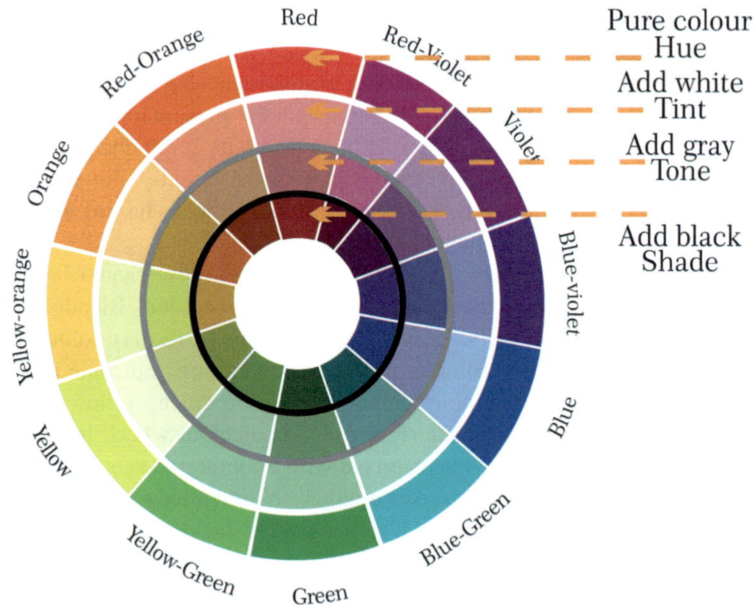

Fig. 3.2 Colour wheel is a resource for choosing colours for a healthcare presentation

Cool and Warm Colours

Colours are often considered as warm and cool (Fig. 3.3). Bright colours like red, orange, and yellow are warm colours; Warm colours stand out and are noticed. Blue, green, and purple are cool ones. Cool colours, especially their dark shades retreat into the background. White and very light colours catch the eye, whereas black and very dark colours generally are less noticeable.

Colours from the same group mix agreeably. Warm colours mix well amongst themselves and with shades of brown. Cool colours blend well with each other and with multiple shades of grey. Delicate colour contrasts do not work well in projections; high colour contrasts are effective in presentations. White, black, grey, and beige are grouped as neutral colours and blend with all the colours. Printed black and white page looks elegant but stark black background and white text slides look boring; substituting yellow for white considerably improves the situation; adding subtle gradient of black and white adds depth to a presentation.

People attribute moods, traits, personalities, and emotions to colours (Fig. 3.4). Colours may be used to project the theme of the matter being presented. However, such opportunities are rare in health care and scientific presentations.

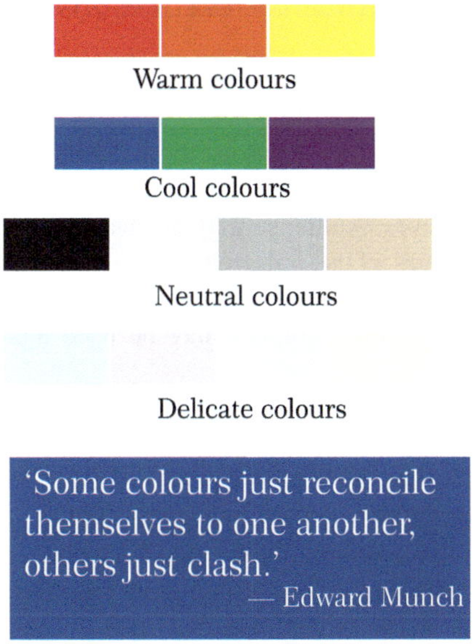

Fig. 3.3 Colour combinations for healthcare presentation

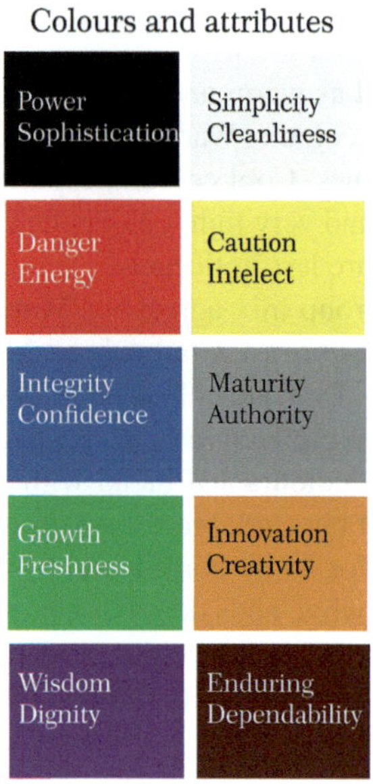

Fig. 3.4 Colours and their popular attributes; 'Colors and emotions are friends'-Anonymous

Colours for Healthcare Presentations

In medical presentations black, white, blue, and grey colours are popular; yellow, gold, and violet are used for special occasions (Fig. 3.5). However, red and green are best avoided; in combinations these colours are jarring to the eyes; eyes have difficulty to tell between these two colour wavelengths; they cause discomfort and easily tire the eyes. Audience may get headache and feel nauseous because their combination gives a false pulsative impression on screen. Bright blue and red make one such unpleasant combination; red and green have similar effect. However, if needed these vibrating colours may be used against a neutral (complimentary) background.

Slides with sharp contrast makes highest impact; for example, dark background and light coloured text or vice versa. Another option is choosing a colour and using its tint, tone, or shade for contrast; using colours from opposite side of the wheel is also an effective strategy; one should select such colours which when used together create maximum visual interest. A different strategy is to choose a tone, tint, or shade of a colour but not its pure hue; next select a pure colour three spaces away on the wheel as a highlight colour. When it comes to number of colours in a slide, less is more; two or maximum three colours suffice in a medical presentation.

PowerPoint and other presentation programs offer colour themes. A theme is a group of specially selected colours that go well with each other. The readymade colour themes offered by presentation programs are fail-safe to use in a presentation

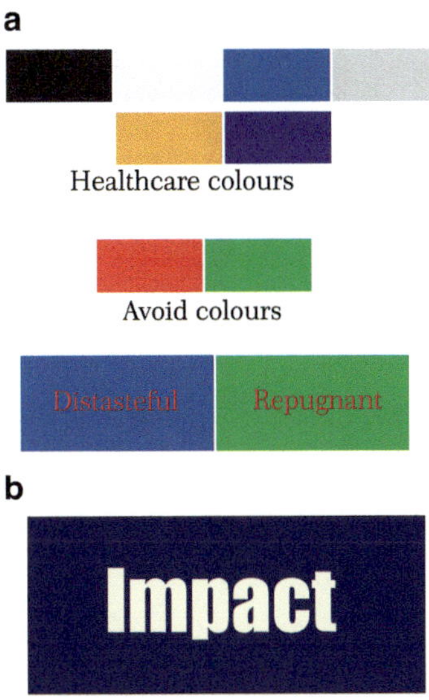

Fig. 3.5 Popular colour arrangements for healthcare presentations. (**a**) an assortment of colours that are useful in a healthcare presentation and a selection of do not use colours for presentation is shown. (**b**) Plain deep blue background and light lettering in bold font makes a definite impression

since most of the healthcare professionals are not trained as graphic artist and do not have the practice of choosing attractive and meaningful colour combinations (Fig. 3.6).

Colours may be used in various gradients, i.e. a colour fades and merges into another. Such colour gradients are often seen in nature; it is nature's way of blending colours. Use of combinations found in nature bolsters maximum appeal and may be used to create attractive backgrounds for the text slides or for shading of text itself. Use of such gradients for text should be limited to large and decorative text; gradients should not be used in normal text.

In a medical presentation, to convey the message effectively one needs to be relevant and stimulating. Use of colour helps, improves learning, and comprehension, when used judiciously.

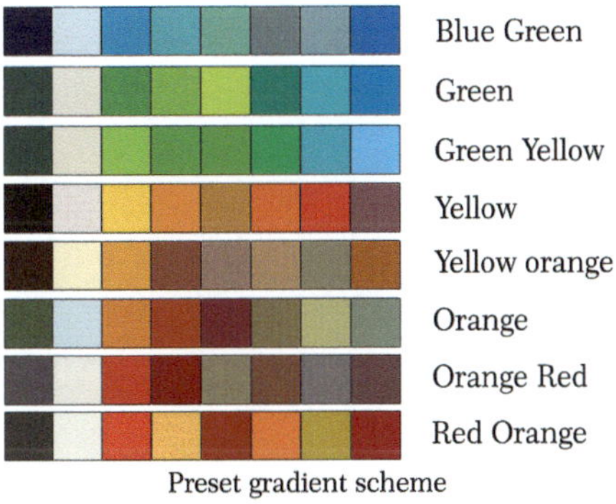

Fig. 3.6 Examples of preselected themes for healthcare presentations

Digital Imaging and Formats

4

Contents

History of Digital Imaging

The basis for digital camera is an image sensor, metal-oxide-semiconductor (MOS) invented by Mohamed M Atalla and Dawon Kahng at Bell Labs in 1959. The use of mosaic photosensors to digitize light signals and produce still images was conceptualized by Eugene Lally in the 1960s while working at Jet Propulsion Laboratory (JPL), a NASA contractor. In 1975, Steven Sasson at Eastman Kodak built the first digital camera. The camera weighed 3.6 kg, had a resolution of 0.01 megapixels and took 23 seconds to form an image. Eric Fossum of JPL in 1990 improved the technology and miniaturized cameras for use on spacecrafts. Later Fossum developed that technology for use in web cameras, dental radiography, automobiles and in camera phones. Similar technology is used in larger digital cameras.

A. J. Thakur, *Tapping the Power of PowerPoint for Medical Posters and Presentations*, https://doi.org/10.1007/978-981-19-1816-2_4

Digital Camera

Digital cameras for medical photography are available since the late 1990s. Cell phone cameras appeared around 2000 and now are very popular. Since 2010, digital point-and-shoot, DSLR, and mirrorless digital cameras are available. All these types of digital cameras generate good images but one has to learn to use these to produce high-quality pictures for medical presentations. This requires specialized training and knowledge of technology and a good presenter should acquire it.

Raster and Vector Images

All the healthcare presentations are now done in digital format. Every picture that one projects is an image file. There are a large variety of formats, and each has special qualities and shortcomings. One needs to choose horses for courses. A right type of file makes a difference between picture perfect projection and out of focus shoddy pictures on the screen. It is worth knowing about image file formats to excel in medical presentation.

Images files may be classified as raster and vector files on the basis of their resolution, the quantum of detail they contain, and where these may be used (Fig. 4.1). A raster image is a digital graphic that is created by placement of pixels in a static grid. A pixel is a smallest unit of information in a digital image. Each pixel is a tiny square made up of 3 sub-pixels, namely RGB (red, green, and blue) that cannot be seen by human eye; the three colours bend into a single tint at the pixel level. A raster image is like a mosaic: When seen from a distance one can appreciate the image; on a closeup it breaks into small squares. The lens of a camera translates the light rays into miniscule coloured pixels that join up to create a genuine digital image.

Raster images are dependent on resolution because each pixel is contributing to the whole; more pixels mean higher quality or resolution of the image because there is more facility for colour blending when seen from far. Conversely, fewer pixels mean when enlarged there will not be adequate pixels to provide continuous shading and the image will breakup or pixilate. Raster images are used in photography and video. Photo like illustrations and large images also use raster file format.

Raster images when formatted, may or may not lose data; lossy or lossless compression depends on how a format handles the image; in lossless formats image reconstruction is reduction of the size of an image without any quality loss. Usually this is achieved by removing unnecessary metadata from JPEG and PNG files. In lossy image formats there is imperceptible reduction of the colour and details; repeated editing noticeably reduces image quality. Lossy files are smaller than lossless ones; advantageous on web viewing and download speed but disadvantageous for presentation. Photoshop, Lighthouse, After Effects, Corel Photo-Paint are a few of the apps that edit raster images.

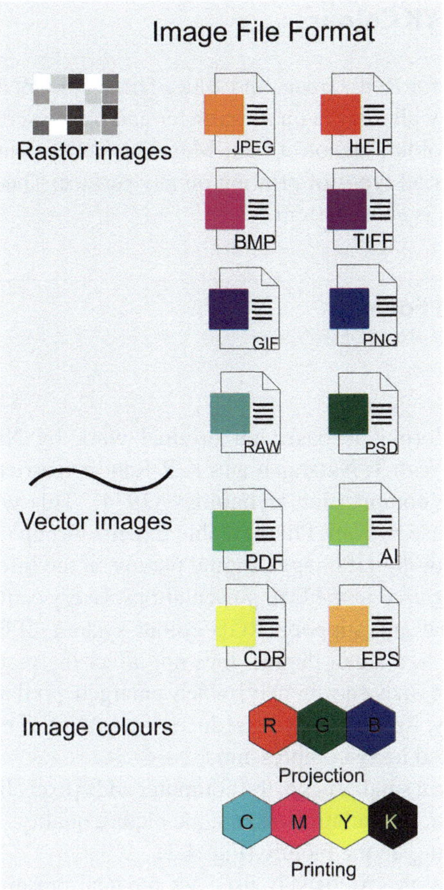

Fig. 4.1 File Formats that support raster and vector images

A vector image is a flexible and scalable digital graphic based on mathematically calculated paths. Vectors are geometric shapes that can be stretched or curved as required. A vector is made up of points, polylines, and polygons. Colour can be added to lines and shapes created by lines. Together a convincing image is created. Vector images are not affected by resolutions. They can be minimized or maximized while maintaining the image quality. Vectors are used in graphics, animated graphics, and precise illustrations. Software like CorelDraw, Illustrator, Affinity Designer, and Inkscape create vector files; PDF is a vector format; PDF files project without pixilation.

RGB & CMYK Colours

RGB stands for Red, Green, and Blue. These colours are used in digital projectors and to display all images on a computer and phone screens.

CMYK colours denote Cyan, Magenta, Yellow, and Key (black). This colour scheme is for all types of printing on any surface. The scheme is not as perfect for projection as is RGB system.

Image File Formats

JPEG

JPEG This format is based on original work by Nasir Ahmed (Born 1940 in Bangalore). With T. Natarajan and K R Rao, he carried out the basic research that led to image compression technology (1974). This was modified and altered for commercial use by Joint Photographic Experts Group (JPEG). This format is extensively used for digital images, digital photos on the Internet, and on social media. It is also widely used in medical presentations. Every camera saves images in JPEG or similar format and supports RGB colour system. JPEG is a lossy raster format; compression to a small degree does not affect the picture quality; steep reduction decreases file size enormously; when enlarged pixilation occurs diminishing the image quality. Repeated saving reduces the quality of image in JPEG format; this is why it is called lossy compression.

To enlarge a small image, the computer adds pixels by approximation to make up the image space; pixelation occurs, the picture quality suffers and one can see small squares making up the picture (Fig. 4.2).

JPEG files are extensively used for medical presentation. One should securely save original JPEG files for future use; copies should be used for presentations. This helps if the material is to be printed at a future date.

HEIF

HEIF (High Efficiency Image File Format) is an image file format is also based on Nasir Ahmad's original work and is similar to JPEG image format but supports animation. It allows superior compression, stores more information, and produces higher-quality animation than GIF with a much smaller file size. Apple phone cameras use a variant, HEIC (High Efficiency Image Container); if needed Mac computers easily convert these file to JPEG.

BMP

BMP—Bitmap file format also known as Bitmap is a simple structure image format for Windows; BMP or Bitmap handles graphics in Microsoft Windows operating

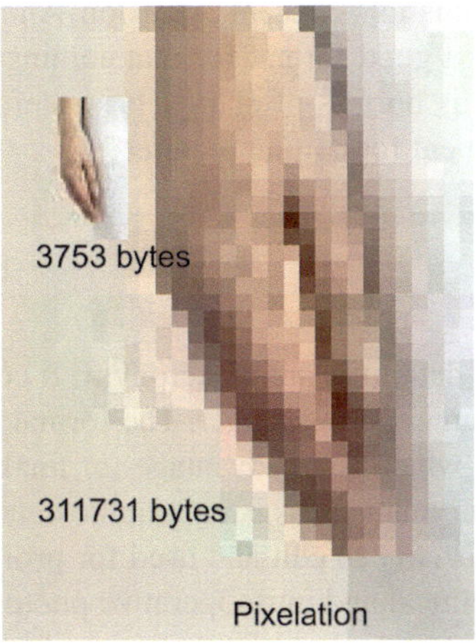

Fig. 4.2 When a small digital image is enlarged, its fineness is lost and square pixels are visible; pixelation occurs

systems and other programs as it is royalty free and simple in structure. These are large in size and lossless compression is possible; lossless compression is possible in ZIP algorithm. Colour spectrum is wide and robust. Files are difficult to handle on email or web platforms because of their large size.

TIFF

TIFF (Tagged Image File Format) is a flexible, adaptable format for handling images and data within a single file. It is a lossless raster format; saved images are of high quality and are often used in photography and printing. This format is also recommended for high-quality scanning. It saves colour better than JPEG. Using this format in presentation makes the file very heavy, slow moving and may lead to computer hanging during a show.

GIF

GIF (Graphic Interchange Format). It has limited capacity for colour. It is suitable for graphics with relatively few colours such as simple diagrams, shapes, logos, and cartoon style images; format supports 256 colours. GIF is also used for small animations in the presentations. It has lossless compression and is apt when only one colour dominates the image. It is a popular format for web images. GIF is pronounced as JIFF or GIFF; the creator Steve Wilhite prefers jif with soft g as in gym.

PNG

PNG Portable Network Graphics was created to replace GIF. It offers better compression and colour capability (true colour [16 million], grayscale, and index colour) but does not support animation; a recent extension, Animated PNG—APNG is making up the deficit. It is a good format for maintaining graphic files as it stores all colours well and there is no loss of clarity. It is useful for large, highly coloured images. PNG is convenient for editing pictures.

RAW

RAW It stands for raw data; it is not an acronym; It contains the unprocessed data captured by a digital camera or a scanner. The format stores processed and unprocessed form separately which is an advantage for final output. These formats store various types of data but main stress is on graphic data. It is used to acquire photographic data. This file is easy to edit and used for professional grade photographic work. It is useful for clinical and intra-operative photography. Needs processing in other softwares like Photoshop and Lighthouse to obtain high-quality photographs. RAW formats exist in under various labels. A few well-known are: CRW (Canon), NEF (Nikon), and DNG Digital Negative (Adobe). RAW format is chosen for high grade clinical and intra-operative photography for images for presentation and printing.

PSD

This format holds design files created in Photoshop app. The data is in multiple layers and is used for image adjustments. It is used mainly to create and edit raster images but can hold vector images too. This file can be exported to several image formats. PSD stands for Photoshop Document.

DICOM

DICOM (Digital Imaging and Communications in Medicine) is a computer language for storing, displaying, and transmitting medical images on scanners, servers, workstations, printers, network hardware, Internet, picture archiving, and communication systems on all imaging devices manufactured by any company. It is also used by hospitals and doctors for seeing the medical images. DICOM was developed in the early 1980s in the USA by National Electrical Manufacturers Association and American College of Radiology and is now used universally. It is used for CT (computed tomography), MRI (magnetic resonance imaging), Ultrasound, X-ray, fluoroscopy, angiography, mammography, breast tomosynthesis, PET (positron emission tomography), SPECT (single-photon emission computed tomography), Endoscopy, microscopy, and OCT (optical coherence tomography). DICOM language is used in radiology, cardiology, oncology, nuclear medicine, radiotherapy, neurology, orthopaedics, obstetrics, gynaecology, ophthalmology, dentistry, maxillofacial surgery, dermatology, pathology, clinical trials, veterinary medicine, and medical/clinical photography.

DICOM includes multiple data including patient name, ID, and image data. It is also capable of storing cine loops and other multi frame data. DICOM images need to be converted to other image formats like JPEG, or BMP, and AVI to be used in medical presentations.

Further Reading

Digital photos for the orthopaedic surgeon. 2004; http://www.indiaorth.org/help/digital_photo.htm

Grollman TB. Digital photography part 1 & 2 handout at electronic skills pavilion American Academy of Orthopaedic surgeon. 2007.

Larobina M, Murin L. Medical image file formats. J Digit Imaging. 2014;27:200–20.

McEnhill P. Making a lecture memorable. Curr Pharm Teach Learn. 2018; https://doi.org/10.1016/j.cptl.2018.04.003.

Richardson ML, Frank MS, Stern EJ. Digital image manipulation: what constitutes acceptable alteration of a radiologic image? AJR. 1995;164:228–9. https://doi.org/10.2214/ajr.164.1.7998545.

Wiggins RH III, Davidson HC, Harnsberger HR, Lauman JR, Goede PA. Image file formats: past, present, and future. Radiographics. 2001;21:789–98.

Supportive Apps

5

Contents

Need for Additional Functions

PowerPoint, Keynote, Prezi, Google Slide, Haiku Deck, SlideDog, and other such presentation programs have several built-in goodies to make refined presentations. The basic functions of these presentation programs have been reinforced with several other supporting tools such as image editing, animations, drawings, video and audio recording, etc. All these add-ons with limited capabilities, do help an average speaker to improve a presentation in several ways. If one wants to excel the average level of the presentation, then a stand-alone program is required for a specific function, e.g. Photoshop for image editing, or Adobe Illustrator for graphics. One should use these and other specialized apps to upgrade the quality of one's presentation

A. J. Thakur, *Tapping the Power of PowerPoint for Medical Posters and Presentations*, https://doi.org/10.1007/978-981-19-1816-2_5

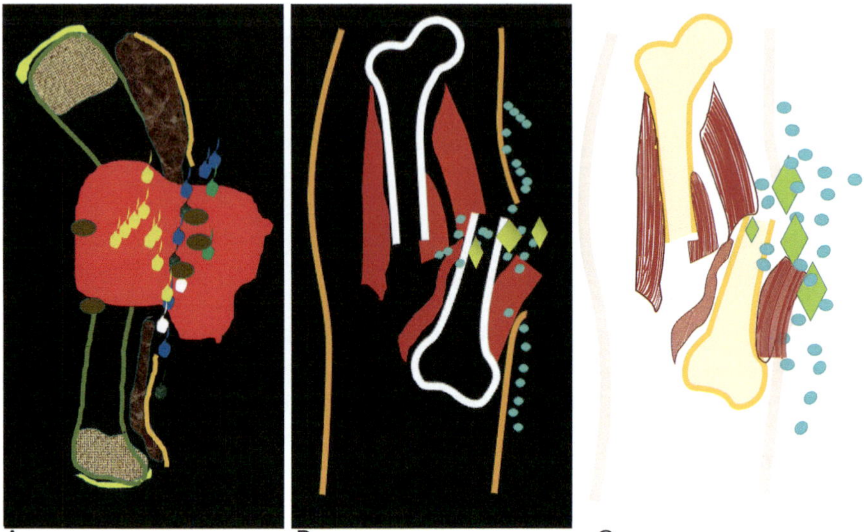

A B C

Fig. 5.1 Graphics in presentation. (**a**) This illustration is made using the basic drawing tools available in a popular presentation program. It lacks the fineness that can be obtained by using a specialized drawing program. (**b** and **c**) are examples; the same theme has been created in two different drawing programs

(Fig. 5.1). However, one has to be proficient in these stand-alone programs as well. A list of such specialized useful accessory apps is included here for quick reference.

Photo Editing Apps

Photo Editor: This free go-to app is simple and easy to use with a friendly interface. It has a wide variety of editing tools in one place and new features are regularly added. Uncomplicated and straightforward to use for editing images.

Adobe Lightroom is an image organization and image editing software. It is a non-destructive editing software that keeps the original image separate from any current edits, saving the edited image as a new file. It is supported on Windows, macOS, iOS, Android, and tvOS. It is compatible with TIFF, JPEG, PSD, PNG, and raw image formats. Its editing functions include white balance, tone, presence, tone curve, HSL, as well as transformation, spot removal, red eye correction, graduated filters, radial filters, and adjustment brushing. Adobe Lightroom is an exhaustive application and has a steep learning curve.

Affinity Photo is a low-cost but resourceful image editor. It is easy to use with a low learning curve. It has been described as an Adobe Photoshop alternative, and is compatible with common file formats such as PSD. It is also a non-destructive photo editor and supports unlimited layers. Its functions include RAW processing, colour space options, live previews as effects are applied, as well as image stitching, alpha compositing, black point compensation, and optical aberration corrections. Affinity Photo is not an image organizer.

GIMP is a free software for photo editing.

Photoshop is the gold standard in this genre. This too has a steep learning curve.

Better Graphics

Affinity Designer is a vector graphics program for macOS, iPadOS, and Microsoft Windows and has been described as an Adobe Illustrator alternative. It is compatible with common graphics file formats, including AI, SVG, PSD, PDF, EPS, and can also import data from Adobe FreeHand files. Its functions include vector pen and shape-drawing tools, vector and raster brushes, dynamic symbols, stroke stabilization, text style management, and vector/pixel export options. It provides non-destructive editing features across unlimited layers, and supports the RGB, RGB Hex, LAB, CMYK, and Grayscale colour models. YouTube has several teaching videos to learn this program for free.

Inkscape is a free and open-source vector graphics editor to create vector images in SVG format. Other formats can be imported and exported. Inkscape can provide vector shapes, e.g., rectangles, ellipses, polygons, arcs, spirals, stars, and 3D boxes and text. It can create vector graphics from photos and other raster sources. Created shapes can be manipulated, e.g. moving, rotating, scaling, and skewing. It has Bezier tool and full complement of text tools.

CorelDraw is a vector graphics program for Windows. It has an economically priced Home and Student version for amateurs that is easy to use and has extensive support on YouTube.

Adobe Illustrator is an app for professionals to produce graphics of very high quality.

Use of a graphic app is very advantageous and a presenter will raise the presentation standards if he or she is able to draw the figures in a drawing program.

Animation Programs

Motion is an app for macOS operating system. It is used to create and edit motion graphics. This is very different from traditional animation software, which requires the use of keyframes to determine the position of an object at any given time. It is difficult to create realistic animations with keyframe mechanism. Motion supports keyframes but has new system of using preset actions which can be combined to create realistic animations.

Open Toonz is an open-source program, easy to use, and good for basic animations. It makes 2D animations. It uses keyframe method and has several function to produce pro-like animations.

Blender is good for 2D animation with powerful drawing tools and a stroke-based workflow. Its grease pencil tool can be used to create beautiful cut-out animations and motion graphics. Blender can also combine 2D and 3D animations.

Adobe Animate

Adobe Animate is a multimedia authoring and computer animation program. Animate is used to design vector graphics and animation for television series, online animation, websites, web applications, rich web applications, game development, commercials, and other interactive projects.

Video Editing

InVideo One can make videos in PowerPoint but it takes much effort and time. Timing the scenes, adjusting them for voiceover content, animations is backbreaking and one often wishes for quicker ways of doing things. Things that are required to be done manually in PowerPoint are done automatically in this program. One can import short individual clips from a long original one. Video correction becomes easy when using products like InVideo. Saves time and effort.

Windows 10 is packaged with the newest version of **Photos app** that is able to create and edit videos with music, text, motion, filters, and 3D effects. Windows Movie Maker is no longer available.

iMovie

This is a free video editing tool for use on iOS devices and Mac and comes with the device. The program has an intuitive interface; it supports very many file formats for video and has an array of editing functionalities. Every version has exclusive modifications to make better videos.

Blender

This video editing free software is a pleasure to use. It has a wide range of animation essentials like UV unwrapping, shading, interface, rigging, and modelling. It is very versatile and lightweight. Perfect for amateur designers, graphic artists, and 3D enthusiasts as it offers quality professional 3D at no cost. Initial learning curve is a bit steep.

Video Converter

Aimersoft Video Converter is an easy-to-use fast app that converts video and audio files between a wide range of video and audio formats, including the popular MP4, MOV, WMV, MKV, AVI, FLV, MP3, WMA, WAV, AAC, AC3, M4A and the uncommon VOB, MXF, TS, ASF, SWF, 3GP, 3G2, DivX, XviD, M4B, M4R, AU, APE. One can edit the video before conversion. It easily transfers the converted, downloaded, edited videos or media files from computer to mobile device. It supports iPhone, iPad, iPod Touch, Android phone/tablet, and external hard drive.

Freemake Video Converter (FVC) is an entry-level video editing app. It can perform simple non-linear video editing tasks such as cutting, rotating, flipping, and combining multiple videos into one file with transition effects. FVC reads the majority of video, audio, and image formats, and can convert these to AVI, MP4, WMV, Matroska, FLV, SWF, 3GP, DVD, Blu-ray, MPEG, and MP3. It rips video DVDs, creates photo slide shows and music visualizations. FVC also prepares videos that can be used on multimedia devices like Apple, Xbox, Sony PlayStation, Samsung, Nokia, BlackBerry, and Android mobile devices. It can also burn compatible video streams to DVD or Blu-ray Discs or upload them directly to YouTube. The basic version is free and higher levels are economically priced—Freemium, Free + Premium configuration.

HandBrake is a free and open-source transcoder for digital video file, which makes ripping a film from a DVD to a data storage device easier. It has a large number of options which makes it difficult for beginners to work; newcomers are advised to stick with the defaults. It is a solid choice as a free video converter and was once voted the most popular app.

Audio Editors

WavePad Audio Editor app is an audio and music editor for Windows and Mac. It lets users record and/or edit music, voice and other audio recordings. It has sound editing functions like cut, copy, paste, delete, insert, silence, auto-trim, and more. It can also amplify, normalize, equalize, envelope, reverb, echo, and reverse audio effects. Speech synthesis, test to voice and voice changer functions are embedded in the program.

GarageBand is an easy to learn free audio editor and built-in audio creation studio inside a Mac device. It can play, record, create, and share audio files. There is an array of realistic amps and effects and a fully-equipped sound library including a selection of drums, guitar and voice presets.

Free Audio Editor is a preferred choice for its simplicity. It has a well-designed interface and supports a range of export formats. Trimming and converting sound files is straightforward. One can digitize sound recordings from rare music cassette tapes, vinyl LPs, and videos and create standard digital sound files. Editing is in the traditional Waveform View or the frequency-based Spectral Display; it has more than 30 native signal and effects processing engines. In Free Audio Editor it is easy to isolate and remove unwanted noise.

Audacity is a free, open-source digital audio editor and recording app. It is available for Windows, macOS, Linux, and other Unix-like operating systems. Audacity can be used for recording audio from multiples sources, and can add effects like normalization, trimming, fading in and out. It is a very popular program in educational field and there have been over 110 million downloads since March 2015.

Text to Speech Programs

Speech synthesis is the artificial production of human speech. A computer uses artificial intelligence (AI) to convert text to speech. Programs now provide high-quality, natural-sounding speech with control of the pitch and speed of the voice.

All these provisions help in generating near normal speech instead of robotic tone from text that can be used in videos. Several text to speech—TTS—programs are available to improve the narration in the presentations.

- Balabolka.
- Natural Text Reader.
- Google Cloud Text to speech.
- Microsoft Azure.

Miscellaneous

Google Input

This app is useful to get text in different languages. Google Input Tools facilitate creating a virtual keyboard interface in different languages. Using it, one can translate/generate an output of words and phrases into any preferred language. Handwriting tool generates typing text by writing with fingers or mouse.

Office Lens

Office Lens uses the device's camera to click a photo of a note, card, or other document. It can capture the image as a whiteboard, a document, a business card, or a photo. This image can be edited and revised by cropping, flipping, drawing, and adding text to it. This is a free app.

Google Lens

Google Lens is an artificial intelligence (AI) based technology that uses smartphone camera and deep machine learning to detect an object in front of the camera, understand it and offer actions like scanning, translation, etc. It can copy a text and make it available for use in the device. It can also search text with Google, e.g. definition of a word.

Perspective Image Correction

Perspective in photography is the feeling of depth or spatial relationship between objects in a photo, along with their dimensions with respect to what the viewer of the image sees. A change in perspective makes objects appear smaller or larger than normal, lines can converge differently; When tilting the camera to take a photo of a tall building from the ground, the building appears to fall away. These distortions are correctible in apps. One needs to select the area for correction and set four alignment points around the object needing straightening; the apps do the rest effortlessly and gives a pro appearance to the photo.

SKRWT —pronounced 'screw it'—is a low-cost all-purpose perspective and lens correction app for iPhotos. It rotates and adjusts the photo's vertical and horizontal planes separately and straightens to make them look more natural and symmetrical. It successfully corrects lens distortions for shots taken with adapters, DLSRs, a GoPro or a drone camera.

Perspective Correct is another easy and intuitive 2D correction option for Android, iOS mobile, and desktop. It fixes distortion and skewed pictures with keystone. It can straighten or correct image perspectives either from the camera or from the photo library. The app is useful, either when shooting with, or correcting from the camera roll.

Essential Skeleton 4

This app is produced by Elsevier and is available free but only for iPhone and iPad. It is useful to get the images of the skeleton. Any bone may be selected and viewed in 3 planes, viz. AP, lateral, and oblique.

Background

6

There is a beauty and clarity that comes from simplicity that we sometimes do not appreciate in our thirst for intricate solutions. — Dieter F. Uchtdorf

Contents

Influence of a Background

Background of a slide is like a canvas for creating a painting. Background makes a lasting impression and should be thoughtfully chosen. All presentation apps provide hundreds of templates with a large variety of backgrounds. All these templates are made for commercial purpose and none is suitable for a medical presentation; designs in the background add clutter and distract the audience's attention from the main subject of a presentation. These freely available templates are poorly designed while a few reasonable ones are overused; one may find several speakers using the same background in a conference; an embarrassing situation. A slide's background need not be decorative but should have a positive impact on the message that is being given out. It is a sound policy to start with a clean sheet and create a simple design for presentation (Video 6.1).

Supplementary Information The online version contains supplementary material available at [https://doi.org/10.1007/978-981-19-1816-2_6].

A. J. Thakur, *Tapping the Power of PowerPoint for Medical Posters and Presentations*, https://doi.org/10.1007/978-981-19-1816-2_6

Projection Method

Modern conferences use either digital projectors or LED flat panel display. Digital projector is an image projector which receives digital signals and projects an image on a screen using a lens system. Present day projectors use powerful LED light source which provides higher lumens than conventional mercury or Xenon arc lamps. As a result, the images are seen even when the meeting hall is not totally dark. LED flat panel display is a new device that synthesizes very bright images. There is no lens or light source; the signals are directly fed into the display panel. This brilliant display can be clearly seen in a large conference hall even with generous ambient light. LED wall offers higher contrast ratios than a projector and is a superior alternative to a traditional projection screen, and is being used frequently for large, clear, and crisp display. However, brightness of LED panel may cause discomfort to the audience in the front rows. When projectors are used the images are paler in comparison to the LED wall; additionally the type of screen on which the image is projected also affects the quality of the presentation. The background colour may be chosen depending on whether the presentation will be projected on a screen or displayed on a LED flat panel.

How to Combine Colours

Red, orange, and yellow are warm colours; green, blue, and violet are cool colours. High contrast between the background and text colour is important to make an impact. The further the colours are apart on the colour wheel the higher the contrast and the better the perception. High divergence makes the text appear to float above the background and not merge into it. Choosing red-violet and yellow-green or violet and yellow creates a complementary colour combination (Fig. 6.1). A split complementary combination is two adjacent and one complementary colour; orange, red and blue; violet, blue and yellow. A triad combination has orange, violet and green or red, blue and yellow. A tetradic has blue, green, orange and red or yellow, green, violet and red. Analogous combination has colours sitting next to each other on the colour wheel like blue, blue green and green or orange, red orange and red. In monochromatic combination tints, tones, and shades of the same hue are used.

How to Build up a Colour Combination

Presenting in a dark room one may use dark background and light text, e.g. Black background and white lettering; it shows the letters in sharp contrast. When using small fonts in this combination, small bright letters appear to spread, merge due to excessive whiteness and readability decreases, especially in the back rows (Fig. 6.2). The adverse effect may be mitigated by using yellow lettering. A better solution to improve readability is to use fonts in 40 points or higher; larger font means less

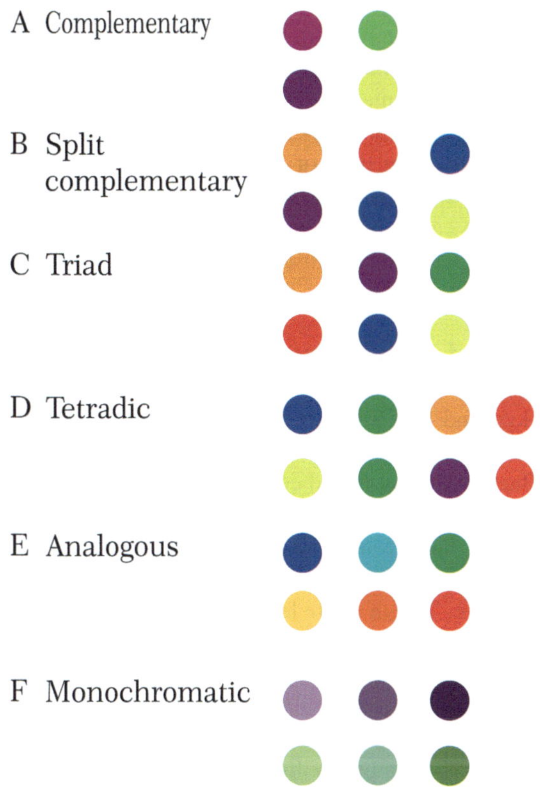

Fig. 6.1 Convention of combining colours. (**a**) Complementary (**b**) Split complementary (**c**) Triad (**d**) Tetradic (**e**) Analogous (**f**) Monochromatic. See the text for details. The groupings shown are illustrations and not recommendations for background colours for a slide

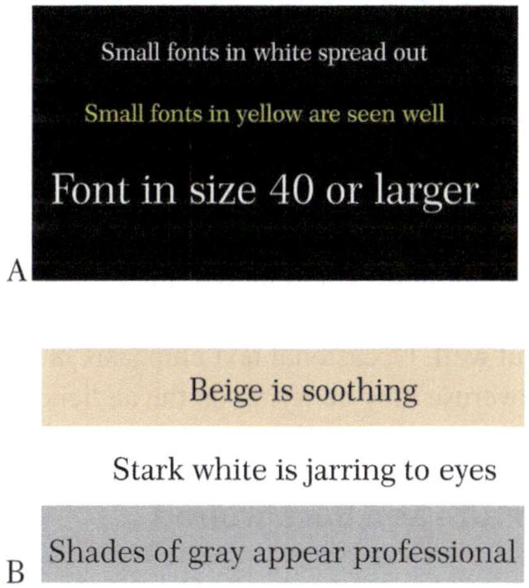

Fig. 6.2 Background genre. (**a**) Dark background (**b**) Light background

material on the slide, which is a good thing. A popular template has a gradient of black and white as the background of a slide. However, black background and white or yellow lettering is not a normal reading pattern; the ambient light is poor and leaves the audience depressed after a long talk.

Light background and contrasting dark shade of text make it easy to read. White background and contrasting black text are an everyday combination seen in a newspaper or a book; however, stark white background is jarring to the eyes and is too plain for a presentation. Light beige or light shades of grey make a professional looking background. Dark text stands out against these backgrounds. In a room with abundant ambient light or when majority of lights are kept on, dark text on light background is well seen. This combination leaves generous amount of light in the room, one can see more in the vicinity, and note taking is easy. Even after a long lecture, it leaves the atmosphere cheerful.

Choice of a Background

Background of a slide may be of a solid colour, gradients of single or multiple colours, a textured background, a picture, or a drawing.

Background of a solid colour makes a constructive impact. In days of cardboard mounted slides, blue was the popular background colour. It was easy to make slides with blue background by using dia-azo chemicals. Blue is a pleasant, calming colour; one feels assured and confident. Colour blue is a well-accepted and a fail-safe choice. Text in white lettering against blue backdrop stands out (Fig. 6.3).

Colour purple makes a regal setting for white letters. Black letters on yellow background look distinctive; all cautionary signs in a radiology department and on the highways have this combination. Colour Orange stimulates mental activity and is suitable for a medical presentation. Green is a restful colour for eyes and is appropriate for background colour; however, lettering should not be in red; choice of white or yellow colour for letters makes a pleasant reading (Fig. 6.4). White is an epitome of simplicity but as a background colour it dazzles, more so when LED wall replaces a projection screen. Solid Black or its gradient is a popular choice when LED flat panel display is used because it cuts down the jarring brightness and is a boon for the front line viewers in an auditorium.

A dark does not necessarily mean black. When needing a combination of dark background and light text, an elegant colour scheme to consider is navy blue or dark purple shade with text in white or yellow. Additional third colour for occasional highlighting a word or two could be red, lime green, camel orange, and light blue. Warm beige makes a decent light background and text in dark blue, black, or dark purple stands out well. Occasional text emphasis in dark green or burgundy fits the scheme but its overuse may be trying on the audience.

Logo and texture as a Background

Use of patterns, natural scenery, or artwork as a background for title slide is often seen but is bad for readability (Fig. 6.5). A presenter may want to use a drawing or an institution's logo as a background. Such a background may not be of a uniform shade and may make reading the text difficult. Background colours may vary from one area to another; a text line may not be visible initially and may suddenly appear

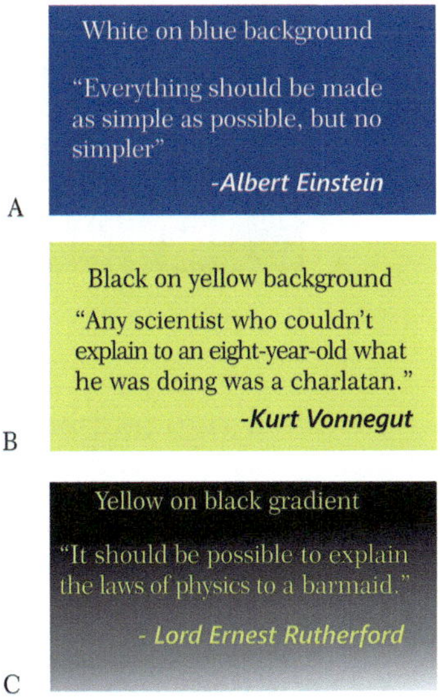

Fig. 6.3 Solid colours make an impressive background. (**a**) Nostalgic blue and white combination of dia-azo era. (**b**) Cautionary signs on roads are in yellow and black because of its high visibility (**c**) Gradient black is a purposive background when LED flat panel display is used

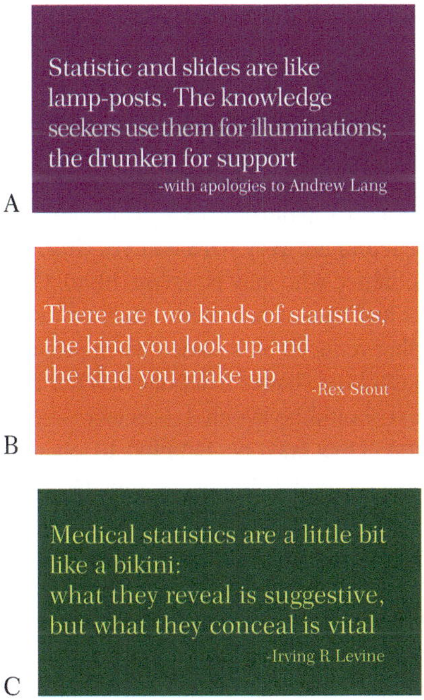

Fig. 6.4 The triad colour scheme—orange, green, and purple—is exceptional. (**a**) purple is associated with rarity, royalty, magic, and mystery. (**b**) Orange symbolizes energy, vitality, cheer, excitement, adventure, warmth, and good health. (**c**) Green is the colour of freshness, hope, and youth

due to change in the background. If one has to use a graphic or a logo, then it should be very subtle; the difference between its lightest and darkest shade in the background should be minimal; use of watermark feature in the app may be useful. A textured background occasionally stands out in a conference. The choice of texture should match the subject of the presentation.

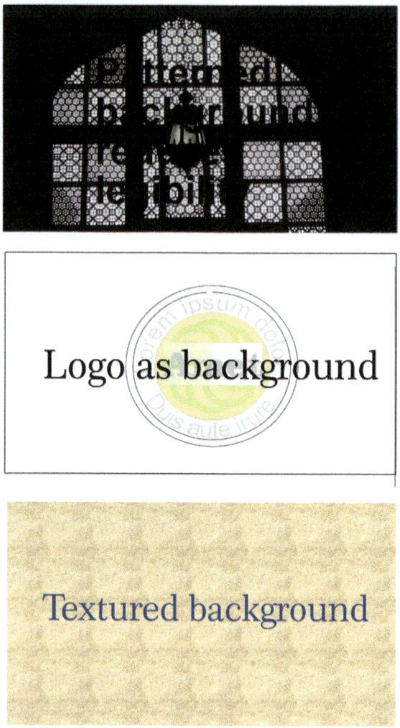

A B C

Fig. 6.5 Other types of backgrounds. (**a**) A pattern in the background may make it difficult to read the text, (**b**) Use of logo as a background has its problems (**c**) A textured background at times becomes the purpose

Colour Combinations to Avoid

Colour combinations to avoid are red-green, orange-blue, and red-blue. Red and green colours clash and are very hard on eyes (Fig. 6.6). They also create problems for 8% of male audience who may be colour blind. Orange and blue appear to vibrate against each other and cause unpleasant effect on eyes. Red and blue have poor contrast which is further reduced on a screen when projected. Another common problem is the inability to tell blue shades from one another and from purple shades. Primary blue colour for text should be avoided. It is unwise to use multiple backgrounds in a single presentation. One may be tempted to change the background to indicate change in focus, but the ploy is too distracting and may be avoided. A sound practice is to use one background for all the slides in a presentation.

Cap the Colours

Limit the number of text colours on any one slide to three. For black background, white, bright yellow, and light orange work very well. For dark blue background white is excellent. Red and black lettering on a yellow background also stand out; yellow needs to be very bright (Fig. 6.7).

People suffering from dyslexia often find high contrast between text and background (such as black text on white background. Use of reduced contrast combinations, e.g. navy blue background and yellow text works for dyslexics and normal vision audience.

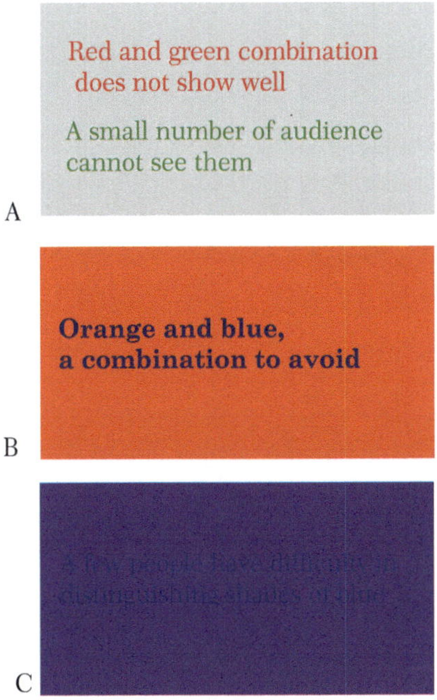

Fig. 6.6 The triad colour scheme to avoid. (**a**) Red and green as colours for text cause problems for many people (**b**) Orange and blue do not go well and may be avoided (**c**) Blue letters on blue background are difficult to read

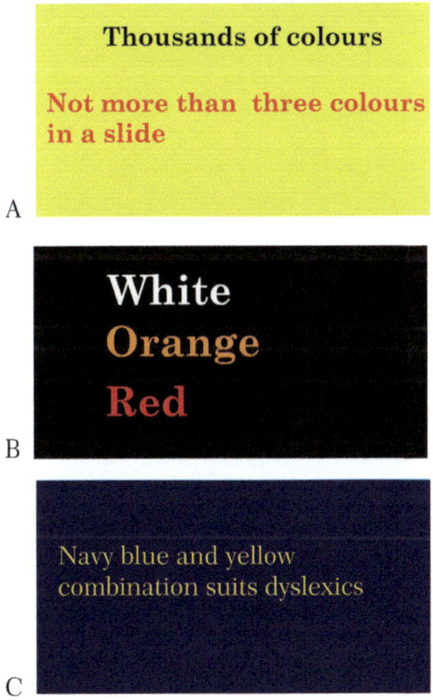

Fig. 6.7 Use of several colours in a slide is not desirable. (**a**) Maximum number of colours in slide should be three (**b**) White, orange, and red text on black background looks impressive (**c**) Combination suitable for dyslexics

The Text Slides

7

'The key to doing text slides right is to remember "less is more" and "bigger is better".' – Anonymous.

Contents

Supplementary Information The online version contains supplementary material available at [https://doi.org/10.1007/978-981-19-1816-2_7].

A. J. Thakur, *Tapping the Power of PowerPoint for Medical Posters and Presentations*, https://doi.org/10.1007/978-981-19-1816-2_7

Introduction

Despite availability of several new gadgets for dispersing information, live lecture still remains mainstay of educational activity (Fig. 7.1). In present context it is impossible to imagine a medical talk being delivered, be it in a conference or a class room, without a supporting computer-based slide show.

The presentation program that runs the slide show, and there are several of these, has 3 main functions. It allows insertion of text and its formatting, it has a way of inserting and modifying graphic images, and a facility to run a slide show to project its contents on a computer screen or through a digital projector on a big screen.

In a medical talk visual material is used to reinforce a strong oral presentation. It is common to project salient points of a talk in text slides. Thus, the text slides are an integral part of scientific presentation as these convey and reinforce thoughts and concepts in visual format. To hear the words and at the same time see them on the screen, makes a lasting impression on the audience. The writing on the screen swiftly impresses the audience.

Text slides are the main stay of a presentation and are appropriate for introducing the objectives of a study, for definitions, summary, conclusions, and are best for quotations. A text slide is catchy if its typography, line spacing, and alignment are appropriate (Fig. 7.2).

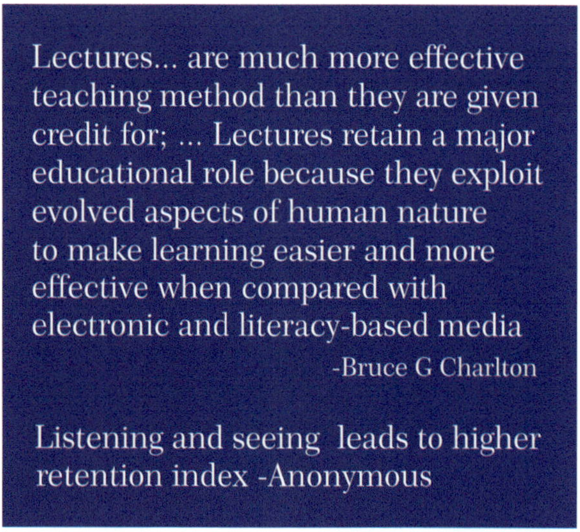

Fig. 7.1 Usefulness of a live lecture in digital age

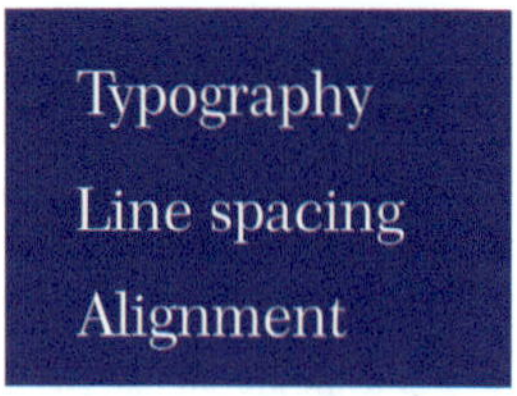

Fig. 7.2 Three design elements of a smart text slide. 'Just like people are often judged by their physical appearance, so will the content be judged by the design elements used—many times even before it is read'.—Anonymous

Typography

Typography in context of a presentation is a technique and an art of arranging letters to make the displayed text clear, simple, readable, and engaging. The word 'typography' in English comes from the Greek roots; typos = 'impression' and— graphia = 'writing'. Typography involves selection of typefaces, fonts (point sizes), arranging the length of the sentences and designing a paragraph. Typography used to be an exclusive domain for compositors, graphic designers, art directors, and specialized artists. The digital age has opened up this controlled zone to lay users. Now anyone who owns a computer now can dabble in typography whether or not having had any training or knowledge of the principles and best practices of the discipline. Such a person may fail to make the best use of easily available computer tools since being unaware of the intricacies of type setting, and may fail to achieve clarity with appropriate selection of serifs, and upper- or lower-case lettering. Such a person's poor understanding of limitations of human vision may lead to poor projection of the message and some people in the audience with vision problems may miss out on the details of a presentation. An uninitiated presenter may fail to achieve the main aim of making a presentation.

Legibility, readability, and aesthetics are central characteristics of typography. Legibility means the comfort with which a reader can interpret a symbol. In presentation the legibility of text depends on the viewing distance; the angle that text subtends on the viewer's eye and a person's ability to see. Age of viewer is important; older adults are disproportionately affected by small text size. Other factors that may affect the excellence of projection are the design of the typeface and the technical grade of presentation medium used.

Readability is the ease with which a reader can follow and understand words, sentences, and paragraphs. Readability is more about their arrangement or even the choice of words. Legibility is a component of readability.

Good legibility and readability improve aesthetics of typography.

Typeface and Font

Choosing a right design for text lettering is important as it can just make or break a presentation. English lettering for computers comes in many designs or 'typefaces'. Each typeface has distinct form and a name. Well-known typefaces are Arial, Times New Roman, Helvetica, Century, Baskerville, and Gill.

A letter under a typeface family may be written in several ways. Variation in thickness of lines gives different look to a letter. Medium, bold, semi bold, condensed, oblique, or a combination like bold oblique are a few examples. This creative variation of a typeface is known as font. Thus, there are several fonts under a typeface (Fig. 7.3).

One may say typeface is the design and fonts are variations of the theme. Metaphorically, typeface is what you see and font is what you use to write the story. Another analogy compares typeface to the name of a Hindu Undivided Family and

Fig. 7.3 Illustration of Serif typeface Century and all its fonts. The terms Typeface and Font are not synonymous. Typeface describes a design of a letter; font is a variation of that design

Typeface	Font	
Century		
	Century 725 cn BT	(Regular Normal)
	Century 751 BT	(Roman Normal)
	Century 751 BT	(Normal, Italic)
	Century 751 BT	(Bold, Italic)
	Century751 No2 BT	(Roman, Normal)
	Century751 No2 BT	(Normal, Italic)
	Century751 No2 BT	(Bold)
	Century751 No2 BT	(Bold Italic)
	Century751 No2 SeBd	(Semi Bold, Normal)
	Century751 No2 Se Bd	(Semi Bold, Normal, Italic)

fonts are family members or co parceners. The modern-day computer users apply these two terms interchangeably; however, these are not synonyms. This confusion between typeface and font (the various styles of a single typeface) occurred in 1984 and is attributed to Steve Jobs. He mislabelled typefaces as fonts for Apple computers; no one corrected his mistake. The computer industry continues to use the term 'font' when the right word is 'typeface'.

Serif and Sans Serif

Typefaces are classified as Serif and Sans serif. Serif is a decorative embellishment associated with a letter (Fig. 7.4). Serif originated from stone carving of letters in ancient Rome. These letters were first painted onto the stone. Brush marks often flared at the corners and at the end of a stroke. As the stone-carvers worked on the brush marks serifs materialized; serifs also helped in sprucing up the ends of the lines as they were being chiseled. In printing technology serif is a decorative stroke or small line at the end of a larger stroke in a letter or a symbol. The letter designs or typefaces that use such decorative stubs are called Serif or serifed typefaces. The designs (typefaces) that do not use such enhancements are without serif- or Sans-serif. Historically, serif fonts can be grouped in 4 types: Old style, transitional, didone, and slab serif. The classification is useful in medical presentation to pare fonts in a presentation.

Serif typefaces have an engaging history. In 1750, Baskerville serifed typeface was designed by John Baskerville (1706–1775) in Birmingham, England. Century typeface was designed in the USA in 1894 for printing of The Century Magazine. The typeface has a high prestige in that country; all briefs for the Supreme Court of the United States are required to be printed in Century family type. In 1931, British newspaper The Times commissioned 'Times New Roman' typeface. This typeface is influential and popular and is often used in book and general printing. Serifed typefaces are popularly used for a large chunk of text forming the main content of a book, magazine, web page, or any other printed or digital work. The serifs or small feet of the letters guide the eyes to the next letter while reading, it is said.

Sans serif means letters are without decorative strokes. (French word sans = without; serif is likely from the Dutch word schreef = line or pen-stroke.) These are letters with less stroke width variation than serif fonts. These are bolder, open type, convey simplicity, minimalism, and modernity; their clarity and legibility are outstanding. Sans Serif letters have taller 'x' height (distance between the baseline and the mean line of lower case letters). The 'x' height of letter is the measure of clarity; the higher the x-height, the more readable a font is likely to be (Fig. 7.5). The Sans Serif letters are taller than in serif typefaces. The sans serif capitals are wide with uniform width. The space between the letters is tight and are less slanted in italic

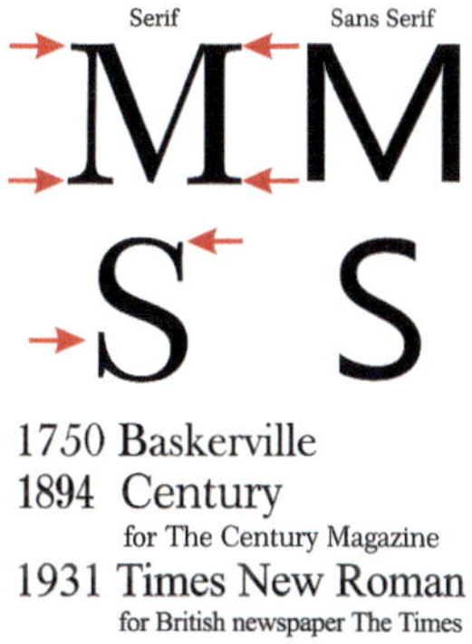
Serif
Sans Serif
M M
S S
1750 Baskerville
1894 Century
for The Century Magazine
1931 Times New Roman
for British newspaper The Times

Fig. 7.4 Serif and Sans Serif letters. Arrows point to serifs, the ornamental extensions to the letters. Three well-known serif typefaces and their year of creation

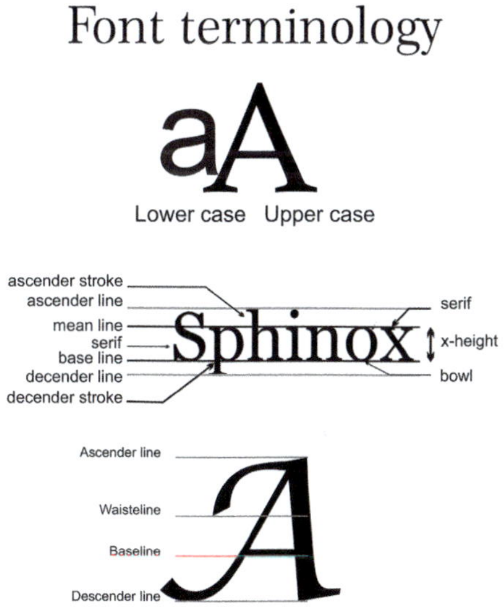

Fig. 7.5 Typography has its terminology

format. These are best used for short text; it is easy to read short text in sans serif typeface in larger size lettering. This is why these are recommended for presentation text in a slide. Sans serif typeface is also popular in large advertisements and for display of text on computer screens. However, in small size sans serif fonts are weak. The most popular sans serif typeface is Helvetica and its variants. It was created in 1957 by Max Miedinger with Eduard Hoffmann and marketed by Hass Type Foundry, a Swiss company. Arial and MS Sans are its clones, created mainly to avoid royalty payments.

Capitalization

Letters may be large or small. Capital letters are referred to as Majuscule. Upper case, capitals, caps, large letters are common synonyms. Small letters are referred to as Minuscule; lower case letter is another synonym. The terms upper case and lower case have a historical background. The movable types for letterpress printing were stored in shallow open boxes called type cases; Cases with capital letters of a typeface were stored at higher level while the cases containing small letters of the typeface were kept at operative height of the work bench (Fig. 7.6). In the current times all the typefaces are available in the computer, but the terminology has stayed and capital letters are called upper case and small letters are still referred to as lower case letters.

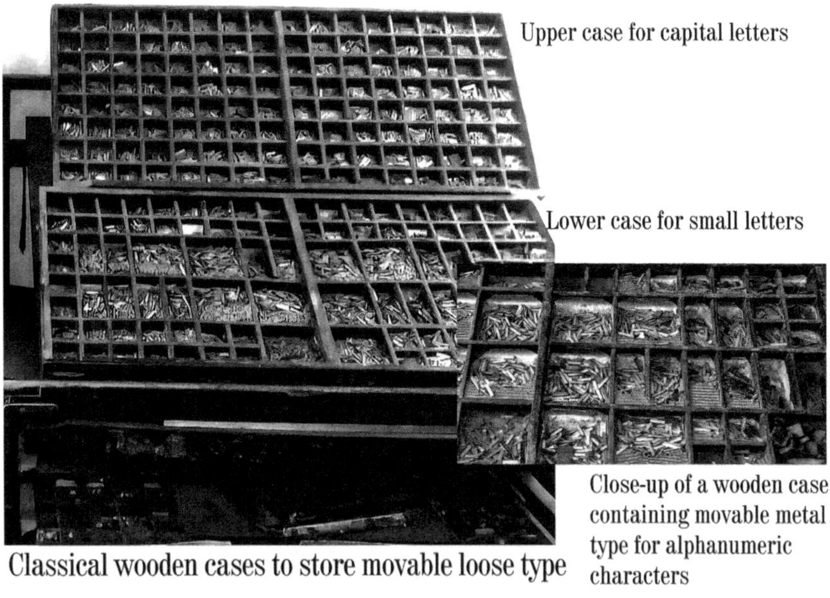

Fig. 7.6 Classical wooden cases to store individual letters cast in metal; capital letters in upper case and minuscules in lower case

Line and Letter Spacing

In a slide presentation adequate distance between individual letters of a word (character spacing) and between words in a sentence (word spacing) enhances its readability, elegance, and lucidity. 'Character spacing' is a function in the presentation programs which alters these attributes. In addition, line spacing—the space between two baselines also affects the readability of a paragraph. Lack of space between the lines gives the text a cramped appearance (Fig. 7.7). The ascenders of the succeeding lines touch the descenders of the previous line. Absence of clear space between lines makes it difficult for the eye to follow from one line to the next. There are no guides or rules for this parameter. The software programs call this facility as leading—reminiscent of type setting by hand when thin lead strips were inserted between the lines to increase the white space. Line spacing or interline spacing is synonymous to leading. Single- or double-line default spacing is a common; other setting options are available as baseline spacing, 50% leading or 100% leading and may be tried and tested for optimum effect. Choice of fonts again affects leading, e.g. serif fonts occupy more area and should have wider line spacing than sans serif.

Case Styles

When entering text in a slide, sentence writing is governed by rules of capitalization, other punctuations, and word spacing to save the reader from confusion; there are several ways of writing a sentence; each one has its identity. The governing practices are called case styles and 4 of these, sentence case, all caps, small caps, and all lower case are in everyday use (Fig. 7.8).

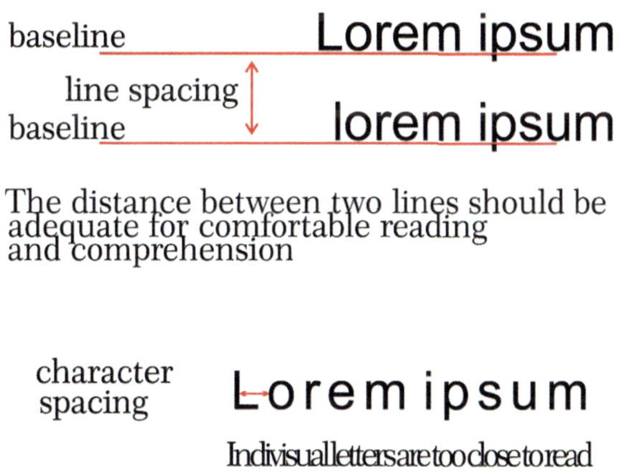

Fig. 7.7 Line and character spacing changes readability of the text on the screen

Fig. 7.8 Text formatting—conventional case style

Case styles

Sentence case

The quick brown fox jumps over the lazy dog

The end of labor is to gain leisure -Aristotle

Whenever I wite a paragraph in English, I first check it with the Google Translator, and most often it says no language detected - M.F.Moonzjer

All caps

(all uppercase)

THE QUICK BROWN FOX JUMPS OVER THE LAZY DOG

IF YOU DO AN OPERATION BADLY, YOU GET BAD RESULT - J SCHATZKER

SMALL CAPS

THE QUICK BROWN FOX JUMPS OVER THE LAZY DOG

EDUCATION IS THE BEST FRIEND -CHANAKYA

all lowercase

the quick brown fox jumps over the lazy dog

apparel oft proclaims the man - william shakespear

Sentence Case

The first letter of a sentence is capitalized and rest are in lower case; this is called sentence case. A sentence case is used in text slides, books, and newspapers. Capital letter at the start of lower case writing helps the reader to identify the start of a new sentence and supports legibility. Audience is accustomed to this type of formatting and finds it easy to read on the big screen.

A capitalized letter is called 'upper case'. Text in upper case is harder to read because all the letters are of the same size, take a longer horizontal space, there is complete absence of ascenders and descenders of the lower case which help in comprehensibility and identification; this is why it takes longer to read all-capital text. All caps case may be used in headings and special situations, such as for typographical emphasis.

In reading sentences and paragraphs, eye recognizes a block of about 3 words at a time and can manage 3 to 4 jumps with ease. More jumps introduce fatigue and errors in reading. The use of all caps renders words indistinguishable as groups, all letters presenting a uniform line to the eye, requiring special effort for separation and understanding. Use of all-capital letters but in a smaller size is called small caps and are used on selected occasions. At times regular size capital letters are mixed in midsentence with small caps to make it look attractive. In engineering drawings usually all caps are used because lower case letters are confusing to read. In Mathematics capital letter denotes higher value than a lower case letter.

When all the writing is in minuscules with no capital letter, it is called all lower case. The style is used for artistic effect. The style is common in SMS language and instant messaging. However, absence of a capital letter may unsettle a reader. In normal use upper and lower case letters are mixed; mixing is guided by grammar of the language or usage of a particular discipline.

Unusual Cases

Use of computer for typography has created a new wave of creativity and given birth to special style of case (Fig. 7.9). These may be sparingly used for panache in a presentation.

Fig. 7.9 Text formatting—special case styles

Special Case Styles

Upper Camel case

TheQuickBrownFoxJumpsOverTheLazyDog

TheSecretOfGettingAheadIsGettingStarted

-Mark Twain

PowerPoint

Lower Camel case

aRistotle iPhone eBay

Snake case

the_quick_brown_fox_jumps_over_the_lazy_dog

rather_elegant_surgical_technique_than_brute_force

SCREAMING_SNAKE_CASE

BREVITY_IN_WRITING_ASSURES_ITS_PERUSAL

Kabab case

the-quick-brown-fox-jumps-over-the-lazy-dog

It-is-part-of-the-cure-to-wish-to-be-cured

Train case

THE-QUICK-BROWN-FOX-JUMPS-OVER-THE-LAZY-DOG

WRITING-IS-A-SKILL-BORN-FROM-PRACTICE.

Studly case

tHeqUicKBrOWnFoXJUmpsoVerThElaZydOG

oPpOrtUnItYfAvoUrsThEPrePaREdmInD

stUdlY cAps NeWs

In upper camel case the first letter of each word is capitalized and spaces and punctuations are omitted. Example is 'PowerPoint'. When first word is in lowercase like 'iPad, eBay and iPhone' it is called lower camel case. In a snake case, the punctuations are eliminated and single underscore is used to separate the words. The same underscore for all capitals is called screaming snake case. Here hyphens are used to separate the words written in lower case. In Kabab case the text written in sentence case is separated by a hyphen. When the sentence is written in all caps and the words are linked with a hyphen, the style is known as train case. The style that does not follow any rules and uses both cases at random, is called studly case; a few examples are: stUdlY cAps, StUdLy CaPs, and NeWS.

Alignment of Text

Text paragraph should be aligned to appear elegant. A text block can be aligned in one of the four ways: flush left, flush right, justified, and centred (Fig. 7.10). Right aligned text is most difficult to read. Flush right is used in Urdu, Persian, Arabic, and Hebrew. In English text slides, it is used to indicate author of a quotation, in formatting numbers in tables, or aligning a text accompanying an image placed on

Fig. 7.10 Four patterns of text alignment: Flush left; flush right; justified; centred

Flush left

This can create a very ragged appearance, particularly if there are lot of long words. With flush-left setting, also called range-left or unjustified setting, each line is filled to the nearest whole word. Letter and word spacing remain constant, so the right hand margin is uneven or ragged.
Hyphenation hardly exits, and when it does occur, it is usually restricted to very long words.

Flush Right

This setting severely reduces legibility. The lines begin at different points, so it will be more difficult for the eyes to find the beginning of each new line. This also has the same raggedness problem and is also harder to read. This style has a use for short captions placed to the left of illustrations

Justified

With justified setting, all lines have the same length and both margins are even,. This is achieved by varying the word spacing, and sometimes the letter spacing too. Most justification methods used by computers also include automatic hyphenation. The shorter the line, the more hyphenation there is. Some word processing programmes lack sophisticated hyphenation procedures. Good hyphenation control is necessary if white island and rivers are to be avoided.

Centered

This can be useful when limited to title pages and short texts, but main text set in the manner is also not so easy to read. Choose one typeface for your main text. For headings within the text, use the same face two sizes larger, or one size larger set in bold. Avoid all the fancy variants like outline and shadow until you are more familiar with the general principles of typography and graphic design.

right side of a slide. Justified text is one where the spaces between words and letters are increased or decreased to align successive lines at both ends; the last line of a paragraph is aligned to one or the other end. Lines where spaces have been decreased are called tight lines, whereas loose lines mean the spaces have been increased. Justified alignment is for long texts in print media. Centred text is also called symmetrically aligned text. It is ranged along an axis in the middle of a column. Jagged starting edges make it difficult to read multiple lines of a centred text. Centred text is the preferred alignment for title of a work, headline, poems, and songs. Central alignment in a slide with just one or two lines of text, improves its visual appearance, grabs viewers' attention, and adds to overall elegance. For short text, centre alignment will be passable. Text should be aligned to appear elegant. Flush left English text is the norm. Centralized text is a fail-safe choice for one or two liner text. In a slide 2 or 3 alignment patterns are appropriate.

Projecting a large paragraph and reading it aloud is a bad idea for any presenter. There is only one thing worse than reading aloud—to point out each word as one goes along. The size of the audience should be considered in planning a slide. In a very large gathering the last row misses out on the details of a text if the size of the letters on the screen is inadequate.

Font Size in a Presentation

Large letters are easy to read and should be used in presentations. It helps people with issues with vision. It also helps people with normal vision who are compelled to sit in the last line of a large auditorium. Size of letters of a font is measured in 'point' which is the smallest unit of measure (Fig. 7.11). In computer writing and in publishing, one point is defined as 1/72 of an international inch. An inch-high letter will be referred to as of 72 points; a font of 24 points is twice the size of a font of 12 points. The default size of letters in popular presentations programs is 28/32 which is far too small for a large meeting. Even for medium or small size meeting, large fonts do not hurt.

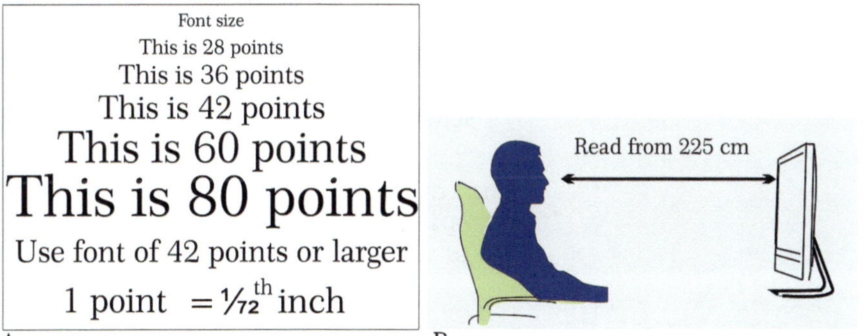

A B

Fig. 7.11 Font sizes (**a**) large font is preferred to ensure legibility (**b**) If a letter is comfortably read at a distance of 2.25 metres from a computer screen, then it is sufficiently large for projection

Text for large medical meeting presentation should never be smaller than 42 points; the larger the font the better the legibility. The title text should be larger than the size of body text by at least 12 points or even more if the space permits. One need not get tied down to a number and may try out a few large fonts and select the biggest that will suit the message. Average size of the font in my presentations is 60.

Choosing and Pairing of Fonts

Pairing of fonts is using different typefaces to draw attention to a message in a slide (Fig. 7.12). A time-honoured pairing is of Sans Serif font Helvetica Neue in the title and serif font Times New Roman for the body text. The high contrast of these two families, one traditional and one modern brings elegance to the presentation and establishes a hierarchy in the message. This combination is usually followed in North America. In other parts of the world there is no established combination. Use of two fonts of a typeface is another conventional pairing. Entirely different appearance and size are effective. A range of such pairings can be worked out for greater visual impact by using typefaces commonly provided in the presentation programs.

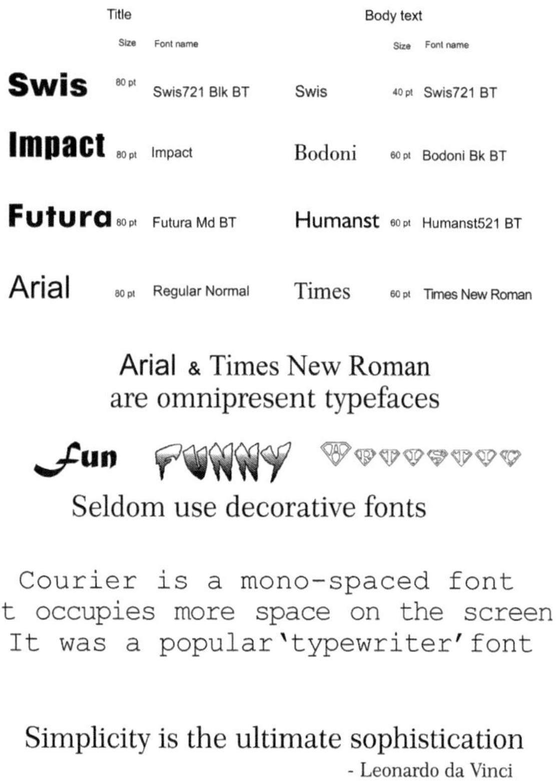

Fig. 7.12 Pairing and use of fonts

Avoid using use more than two typefaces in a slide; very rarely there may be a need for use of a third typeface. Those speakers who travel the globe should stick to two typefaces; Arial and Times Roman; these two are universally available on all computers, from Mumbai to Moscow.

'Regular' or upright lettering is preferred over italics, the slanted one. Outline and shadow styles are best avoided: they have an amateurish look about them and are hard to read. Fun, funky, and artistic fonts are fine for emphasis but not as the main font in the presentation. Type-writers of yesteryears used mono-spaced fonts. These fonts occupy more space on the screen. These are harder to read as our eyes expect the spaces between alphabet letters to change. Keeping the space between each letter of the same size breaks the flow of the characters and makes one's eyes work harder to transmit the information to the brain. These fonts were popular as D.I.Y fonts for those who did not have access to a medical artist. Presently these are used only for special effect. After making the selection of fonts one should look at the them from different distances and in different sizes and ask before the final choice: are they legible and easy to read when used alone and when paired together? Underlining reduces readability by eliminating the recognition effect contributed by the descending elements of letters. Avoid use of Underline feature to emphasize your point.

When needed use Bold or Bold Italic feature; use of colour may serve the same purpose.

Animation of text should be avoided. Zooming words, moving text, letters flying out from the corner of the screen are distracting and difficult to read. If one must use animation, then the effect, 'Appear' is grudgingly tolerable. Dyslexics find it difficult to read serif fonts; they are comfortable with sans serif fonts; typeface Comic Sans is a favourite with this community.

Design of a Text Slide

In the era when scientific community used mounted slides for presentation, it followed the '6-7-7-rule'; It was, six words in a title, seven words in a line, seven lines in a slide. The rule served a purpose of economy, because each slide was made by a long process starting with preparation of the visuals by an artist, photographing the art work, developing the camera film, second processing to give it a blue or red background, putting the celluloid film in a cardboard or plastic mount before it could be shown. All this took time and money. There was need to make optimum use of space available on the slide. '6-7-7-rule' supported the objective. In present times, computer-based presentation programs allow everyone to prepare as many slides as required, very speedily and without incurring any extra expense.

New dictum is one idea per slide (Fig. 7.13). A speaker can present only one thought at time. A single sentence on the screen attracts 100% audience attention. It is unnecessary to have 7 sentences on the screen; seven slides with a sentence each at no extra cost and a little effort makes greater impact. The new rule is 6 words in title, 7 words in the body. The title line of a slide should be short; six to eight words, no more. The body text line should be up to 7 to 10 words, maximum. Every slide need not have a title line; a repetitive title line may be eliminated so the body text dominates.

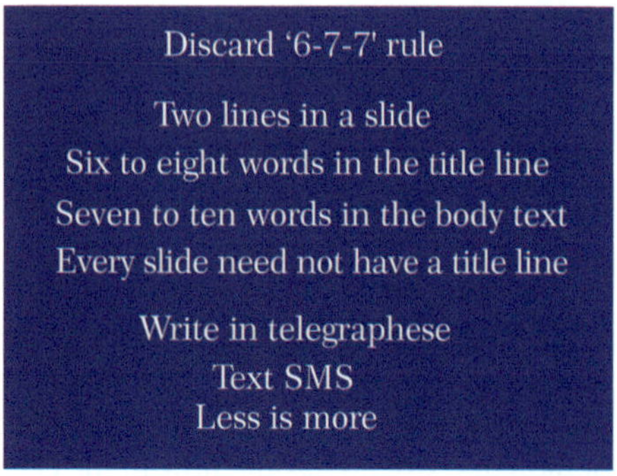

Fig. 7.13 Suggestions to build a text slide

The text in scientific slides should be written in telegram style or in contemporary terms texting in SMS style. It is a tidy way of writing with eclectic words and packs information into smallest possible number of characters. Abbreviations may be used but definite or indefinite articles, punctuations, and other filler words are dropped. A telegraphic sentence is compact, typically containing five words or so. The average length of a telegram message used to be 11 words; 50% of those messages were of 10 or less words.

The text in each slide should be restricted to about 60 characters or an absolute maximum of 120. Characters mean letters, punctuations, numerals, and spaces. An average word in English consists of six characters, with medical texts going up to eight characters. A word slide should have an optimum of about ten words, with 20 words as maximum (Video 7.1). Word slides are often improved by being only partially explicit, requiring the presenter to provide the missing links. This makes the audiences interact with the presenter and slides, because they need the presenter for complete comprehension. Slides designed with this in mind make enduring impression.

Content of a Text Slide

Text contents should be simple. Simplicity has to be worked at and achieved. In fact, this is the work. A simple design takes time to evolve. Simplify at all levels. Avoid repetition of words and symbols. Check every line, letter, dot, dash, and symbol. Always ask, 'Is this necessary'.

In presentation, simplicity is a powerful tool. Slides with title and just one point in the body of the slide have maximal impact; multi-liner slides with several bullet points are commonplace but large paragraphs are ineffective and rare.

Simplicity does not mean bland (Video 7.2). One may add a bit of sparkle with a statement by statement 'progressive disclosure' text slide. These slides allow synchronization of verbal and visual presentation and will often optimize the net effect of the audiovisual communication between a lecturer and his audience.

Avoid use of printed material as an artwork for a slide in a presentation (Fig. 7.14). It is tempting to photograph a text box or table from printed source and use it in a presentation. This should not be done because in printing format, attempt is made to

Table 2-4 2014

Polymers In clInIcal use

Polymers	Degeneratlon tlme ln months	ApplIcatIons	CommercIal product
Poly (lactIde)	6 to12	Orthpaedlc surgery Oral and MaxIllofaclal surgery	FIxsob® (screws, nalls, plns) NeIfIx® (screws, nalls, plns) Arthrex: Blo-Tendesls® Interference screw. Blo-corkscrew® suture anchor LInvatec: SmartScrew® SmartNall® SmartTack® SmartPln BloScrew® ZImmer: Blo-statak® (suture anchor) bone cement plug, prosthetlc stent
Poly (glycolIde)	> 24	Orthpaedlc surgery General surgery	Bloscience: Blofix® screws Dexon® sutures, mesh Bondek® suture Valtrac™ anastomosls rlng, prosthetlc stent
Polycaprolactone	> 24	Drug delIvery Sutures	Capronor EthIcon: Monocryl
Poly (D,L-lactlde-co-glycolIde) Poly (D,L-lactlde-co-glycolIde 85/15 Poly (D,L-lactlde-co-glycolIde) 82/18 Poly (L-lactlde-co-glycolIde) 1090	5 to 6	Sutures Drug delIvery Maxlllofaclal surgery General surgery Orthopaedlc surgery	Polysorb™ Makar: BIologIcally QuIet™ Interference Screw,suture Blomet: Lactosorb® plates, screw, Staple 85/15 mesh, plns, anchor surgIcalclip, VlcrylMesh Vlcrylsuture, Sulzer: PhusIsIIne® Interference Screw Sysorb Screw (50/50) ResorPln® 70/30
Poly (L-lactlde-co-D,L-lactlde) 98/2 Poly (L-lactlde-co-D,L-lactlde) 50/50 Poly (L-lactlde-co-D,L-lactlde) 70/30 Poly (D-lactlde-co-D,L-lactlde-coL-lactlde)	12 to 16		Gelstllch blomaterlals Macrosorb System (Screw, plates, mesh, nall, plns 70/30) Polypln® ZImmer : Leadfix BD Blosclences-No clInical approval BD™ 3D OPLA® (Open-cell Polylactlc acld) scaffold
PolydIoxanone	> 24	Orthpaedlc surgery General surgery	Ethlpln Orthosorb™, Suture mesh folls Bone cement plug
Poly (D-L-lactlde-co-caprolactone) 65/35	24	Nerve regeneratIon	Neurolac® Polyganlcs B.V., Gronlngen, The Netherlands
Polycaprolactone-based polyurethane			TIssue reInforcement Torn tendon replacement patch Interposltlonal space ln osteoarthrltls Artelon® sportmesh™ Arteleon® CMC
LactIde co caprolactone		To prevent adheslon	Mesofol

Fig. 7.14 Printed matter is unsuitable as artwork for a slide

put in maximum information in the smallest space. In a presentation slide it is just the opposite; one prefers to see on the screen a few words and plenty of white space. A slide showing photographed printed text makes a poor impression and may be avoided. Besides, printed material is useless as an art work. It is usually in portrait format. It has too many things on it and is unsuitable for direct photography. Slides should be made in Landscape format with a ratio of 4:3 or 9:16 of height and width. Most computer programs offer a choice of these formats. The projection screens are normally wider than they are high; horizontally oriented slides are preferred.

Lexical Correctness in Medical Presentations

Often it is said, 'The official language of science is not English—it is bad English'-Anonymous. The quote is not to be taken seriously and one should strive to get the correct grammar and spellings in a presentation. Lexical correctness is correct grammar, correct syntax, and correct style.

'Grammatical correctness, after all, has a powerful symbolic value: getting your language right implies that you can obey rules and have systematic approach to science'. —With apologies to Michael Swan. Correct grammar means accuracy of spellings, good choice of word, and proper use of tense, tone, and tenor (Fig. 7.15).

It is in personal interest that a presenter should make every effort to spell correctly. Even small mistakes create a lasting poor impression; A spelling error will stop audiences from reading. They might also assume when there are spelling mistakes, there might be technical mistakes in the presented research. They might even think that the presenter is a bad writer, and therefore, a bad presenter. The trouble caused by spelling errors far outweighs the effort required to correct them. Use of spell check on one's text slides is mandatory. However, a spell check program can eliminate only 95% of errors; no computer will distinguish between their and there, plain and plane, and mail and male. The spelling 'Achilles' (tendon) changes when it is it is written as tendo Achillis; software programmers have yet not caught up with the finesse of English language. Occasionally even a misplaced hyphen can change the meaning, e.g. 'Six monthly doses vs six-monthly doses'. A good

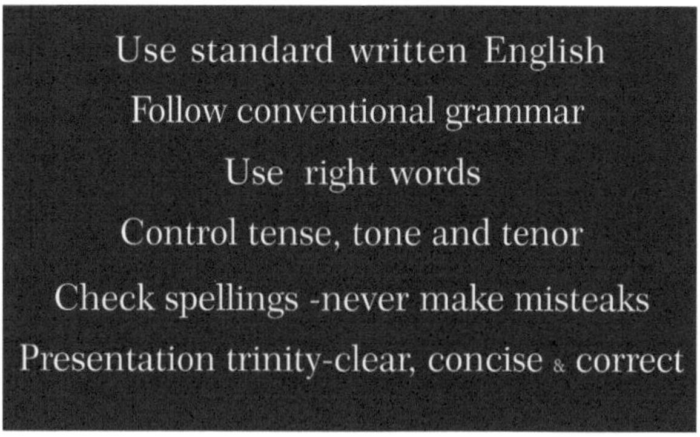

Fig. 7.15 Essentials for appropriate text in a presentation

presenter should manually check the written material on the screen. For want of correct grammar and spellings, a presentation's credibility should not be lost. On occasions, one realizes a spelling error only while delivering the talk. One should not apologize from the lectern for such an inadvertent lapse; 90% of the audience misses it; another 9% notice it but understand it as an error of checking; only 1 or 2 people may point out the lapse. Such people could be handled as necessary nuisance.

Syntax in presentation refers to the way in which words and sentences are placed together. There are set of rules that helps readers and writers to make sense of the sentences. The aim being to help them in putting 'Best words in their best order'. Appropriate syntax makes a presentation stand out. Style in writing is about proper use of punctuation, capitalization, italicization, hyphenation, typography, line spacing, and alignment. Grammar and spelling in a scientific presentation should be flawless. 'Grammar is to a writer what anatomy is to a sculptor or the scales to a musician. You may loathe it, it may bore you, but nothing will replace it, and once mastered it will support you like a rock' says B. J. Chute. In a presentation, important 'Cs' are clear, concise, and correct (Video 7.3).

Use of SI Units

In scientific presentation, the International System of Units (SI) is used. In this context a letter has different meaning when it is written in a lower case or in an upper case.

thus

- 1 s is one second.
- 1S is one siemens.
- 1Sv is one sievert.

There are 7 base units; five of them are written in lower case.

- second for time as s.
- metre for length as m.
- kilogram for mass as kg.
- candela for luminous intensity as cd.
- mole for amount of substance as mol.

Remaining 2 base units are named after people and are written in capital case. Unit of electric conductance is 1S and is named after Werner von Siemens; however, when the same is spelt out, it is written as one siemens in lower case. Unit of ionizing radiation dose is 1Sv which is named after Rolf Maximilian Sievert and is written down as a common noun in lower case as 'one sievert'. Unit should never be made plural. How often have we seen the misuse of the abbreviation for grams, it is not gm, G, or gms but just g (Fig. 7.16).

Fig. 7.16 Symbols and numerals in a presentation

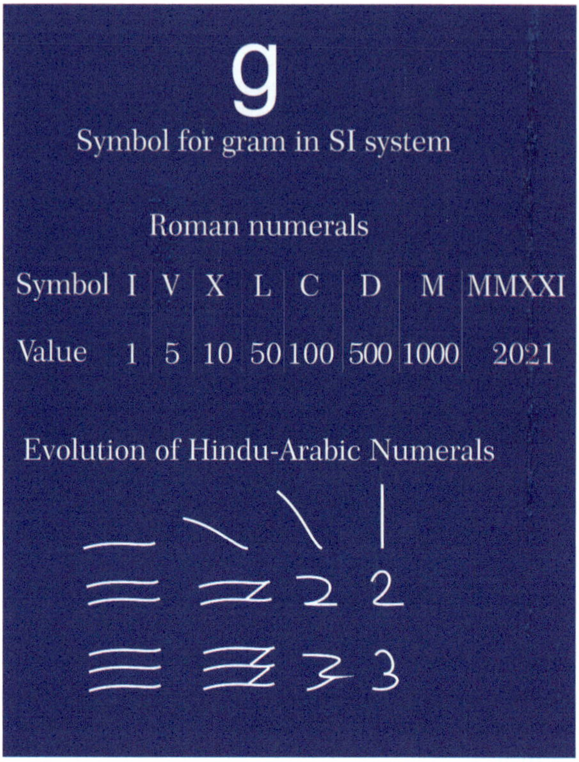

Handling Numbers in a Slide

Roman Numerals

Roman numerals are best avoided in a presentation except when these are a part of established nomenclature. Here are a few instances when use of Roman numerals is appropriate:

- With proper names: Paul Tornetta, III.
- For stating cancer stage but for histologic grade of cancer use Hindu-Arabic numerals.
- Stage IV Grade 2.
- ECG terms: Standard (bipolar) leads I, II, III, s wave in lead III.
- Schedule II drug.
- Enzyme names: HincII.
- Coagulation factors: factor VIII, factor XII.
- Chromosome rearrangements: II bivalent, IV quadrivalent.
- Cranial nerves: Cranial nerves III, IV, and VI are responsible for ocular movement.

Evolution of Hindu-Arabic Numerals

Use Hindu-Arabic numbers*** in a presentation especially in tables. While presenting a list of items one may use numbers only if an order of preference is to be conveyed. If this is not the case, then it is prudent to use bullets while listing.

***William Darrach Halsey, Emanuel Friedman (1983). Collier's Encyclopedia: With Bibliography and Index, Volume 2, Ed. Bernard Johnston (M.A.) ISBN 0029425484, 9,780,029,425,480.

The word 'number' is treated differently in different circumstances. In text, it is best to write full form, but in tables it is abbreviated as No. In statistics its abbreviation 'n' means different things when the case changes; N means total population while n is a sample or response population. A date is written without the suffix, 'rd', 'st', 'th', and 'nd': The subject was given 4 units of blood on 24 July 2020.

Capitalize all designators when combined with a Hindu-Arabic numbers. Some examples are: Day 1, Factor 2, Fig. 3, Group 4, Page 5, Part 6, Phase 7, Sect. 8.2, Series 9, Study 012, Subject 30, Table 3, and Week 14.

The cardinal numerals express quantity like one, two, three, fifty, etc., are written in words. At the beginning of a sentence, or in a title, cardinals are spelt out: Five of 7 dogs remained on the study. Ninety-six subjects were enrolled in the study.

The ordinal numerals express degree, quality, or position in a series, as first, second, and third. Ordinal numbers, first through ninth are spelt out; higher ordinal numerals are expressed in Hindu-Arabic numerals, e.g., 10th, 12th, and 22nd.

The raw numbers and percentages should agree: 'More than 60% (40/79) used the guidance correctly'. Either the percentage or the raw numbers in the example are wrong.

Comma Sutra: Use of Comma with Numbers

Use commas only in numbers longer than 5 digits or more, e.g. 3,255,783; 252,123; and 15,333. No comma is used when numbers are in a table. Large numbers are written as 2.7 million or 2.7×10^6. 'The budget deficit is expected to reach to Rs. 1 trillion (10^{12}) by 2025'.

'You have to design your slides keeping in mind the people sitting in the back of the auditorium. If your slides aren't visible and legible, then you might as well leave them at home'.-Anonymous.

Further Reading

Byfield B. Choosing fonts; 2016. isbn:978-1-921320-47-7.

Data Presentation: Use of Tables and Graphics

8

Contents

Data in Healthcare

In an era of evidence based medicine, data is an important factor and needs to be presented in a manner that is quickly understood by the audience. This requires knowledge of different data display patterns and their minutiae to make an impressive presentation.

Data is collected during field work of a research project by means of questions, systematic observations, imaging, and laboratory tests. Data in its raw form is meaningless. It needs to be converted to information by minimizing, processing, and organizing. Processed data—information can be used for evaluation, planning, and decision making.

Data is of two types: Numerical or quantitative; and descriptive, categorical, or covering frequency of an event, collectively known as qualitative.

Numerical or quantitative data is of two types: Discrete: Full numbers, e.g. in patients in a hospital may be 224 or 225 but not in between these two numbers.

Supplementary Information The online version contains supplementary material available at [https://doi.org/10.1007/978-981-19-1816-2_8].

A. J. Thakur, *Tapping the Power of PowerPoint for Medical Posters and Presentations*, https://doi.org/10.1007/978-981-19-1816-2_8

Continuous: may take any value, e.g. weight 70.5 kg or height 1.8 metres; value can be expressed in decimals.

Descriptive, categorical, or frequency related data are collectively called qualitative. It is arranged in categories based on their quality; there is a gap between two values, e.g. name, religion, marital status. Qualitative data may be considered under 4 heads.

1. Nominal data is distinguished only by its name, e.g. name, sex, or age. Dichotomous data is a nominal data that fall in 2 groups: male/female, rural/urban.
2. When categorical data can be placed in meaningful order based on its quality, it is called as ordinal data. Pain can be classed as mild, moderate, or severe; scores in an examination may be classified as A. 70% and above, B. between 60 and 69%, and C. 50 and 59%.
3. Interval scale data like ordinal data, can be placed in a purposeful order. Interval data, also called an integer, is defined as a data type which is measured along a scale, in which each point is placed at equal distance from one another. Interval data always appears in the form of numbers which cannot be multiplied or divided; however, these can be added or subtracted. The examples include temperature, date, location in coordinates, direction measured in degrees. Example of an interval data is the difference between 90 °Centigrade (C) and 80 °C is same as 40 °C and 30 °C.
4. Ratio scale is the estimation of the ratio between a magnitude of a continuous quantity and a unit magnitude of the same kind. It has the same properties as interval scale. Most biomedical variables form a ratio scale, e.g. weight in grams or pounds, time in seconds or days.

Patterns for Data Display

Data should be presented in an attractive way to create interest in audience's mind; it should be in a compact and simple form so the conclusions may be drawn only by viewing. It may be presented as table or graphics (Fig. 8.1).

People are generally weak at understanding data. Visualization makes it easier for the audience to understand and recall it. One should choose the type of graphic most suitable for the variables concerned (see Fig. 8.9). There are numerous alternatives. A graphic is a very effective tool to summarize information so that its significance can be grasped, literally at a glance. The uniformity in layout, i.e., use of same design and labelling in all related charts or diagrams, helps the audience to reach rapid orientation and understanding.

Effective communication and legibility are prime virtues of a figure for presentation. The presentation software provides very fancy designs of all these figures and multiple effects of text. The figures with shades and fancy text may be very appealing to a creative presenter, but the audience often finds it difficult to follow and at times the data is distorted. A design implemented properly is imperceptible because it supports communication; design improperly done draws attention away from the data and raises doubts about author's credibility. A graphic should be used to inform

Fig. 8.1 Nature of Data and relevant tables and figures for effectual display

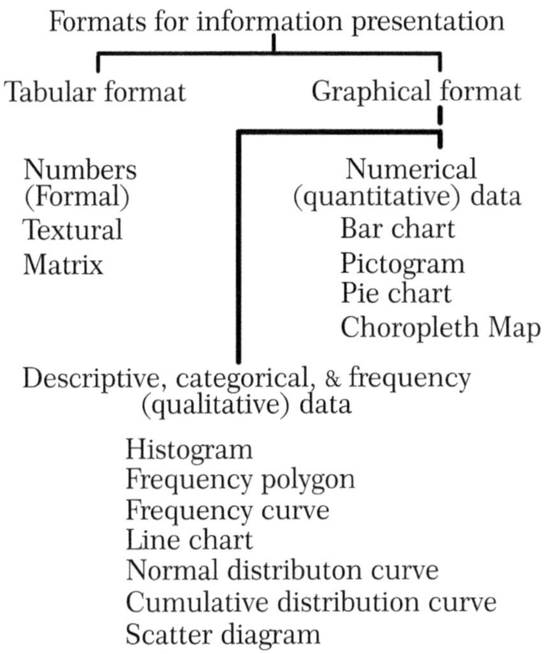

and not to justify William Rushton's statement: The goal of this presentation is to impress, rather than to inform.

Tables and Graphics

Tables

A table displays data and text to support the main topic of a presentation. It is a powerful visual reinforcement when comparison of precise individual values is needed, or values of multiple units of measure are to be displayed. Three types of tables are used: formal table has numerical data in columns and rows; A textural word table displays words, phrases, or sentences in a list form to emphasize key points and summarize information (Fig. 8.2). The third form of table is matrix which is a tabular structure that uses numbers, short words, or symbols to provide visual image of a tabular form.

A table for a scientific presentation has 5 elements: a title—brief, specific, descriptive; column headings, with unit of measure if indicated; row headings in the left-most column to label the rows of the table; body of the table displays the data in cellular format. Table cells contain numerals, text, or symbols; it may not have blanks spaces; missing data may be represented as number 0, abbreviations NA (not available or not applicable), or ND (not determined). Totals and percentages in a table must be verified for accuracy. All the data entries should be aligned horizontally and vertically. The fifth element, a foot note may be used only exceptionally to

Mean functional outcome scores over time in tibal fractures

	Mean SD-44	p-value
Baseline	55.34	
6 months	42.49	0.0001
1 year	47,44	0.0001
5 years	53.78	0.0007

A

Treatment methods according to stage of infection

	Infection	Treatment method	Outcome
Agashe, 2019	1 stage II	Nail retain+ antibiotics	All healed
Menon 2015	4 stage III	Nail retain + antibiotics	All healed
Chitale 2020	1 stage II	Nail removal+ antibiotics	Healed
Lahiry 2014	1 stage III	Nail removal + antibiotics+ debridement	Amputation

B

Objectives of proposals to reform nursing training

Objectives	Report year 1975	1995	2003	2015	2020
Address nurse workforce needs	x	No report	x	x	No report
Address change in nature of illness burden	No report	x	No report	x	x
Increase quality and standards of nursing care	x	x	x	x	x
Cope with expanding knowledge base	No report	x	No report	x	x

C

Fig. 8.2 Tables are of 3 types. (**a**) Formal table, (**b**) Textural table, (**c**) Matrix

bring out an important point. Only standard symbols and abbreviations may be used in tables, e.g. N for number, > for greater than, and % for percentages; WHO for World Health Organization, UNICEF for United Nations Children's Emergency Fund, and EU for European Union. Avoid using lesser-known abbreviations like GOK for God Only Knows or TGH for To Go Home.

Contents of a table for presentation are different than one for publication. A reader of a printed article has unlimited time to study all the data in a table; data can read over and again and compared; data could be appraised at one's convenience and speed. In a meeting the audience gets a passing glimpse of a table; they do not have the luxury of reading at their speed or reread the table if desired. Research data is a result of long hours of hard work and is often voluminous. It is seldom necessary to tell all the details of the method to the audience; the place for such information is not an 8-minute talk but a written communication in some form. The listeners are often interested in the final outcome and want to know that in short. The information in a table must be arranged logically and clearly to validate the central subject of the presentation.

A presentational table should have limited data. It is pointless to copy-paste a table from statistical software; such a copy does not work in presentations. Software generated tables have lines to mark the cell in the table or grid lines in background. Lines create visual clutter and decrease the impact of the vital numbers and text. Removing the cell lines and grid lines adds to empty spaces on the screen making the text and numbers more prominent. A presenter should display only that chunk of the data that maintains audience's interest; this requires ruthless editing and selection. A table should be designed to enable the audience to read it with ease and speed. One should create a table rather than using software generated table template.

Tables require audience's engagement of a higher degree; one can get a focused or disinterested audience; an engaging design of the table is helpful to keep them focused. A presentational table may not have more than four columns; no more than seven rows; the row count starts from the title line, includes column headings, row headings, and if present, even the foot note (Fig. 8.3).

7 ROWS

1	Charnley cemented acetabular component			
2	radiographic loosening at 20 years			
3	Author	Hip	Revision	Loosening
4	Wroblewski 1992	57	-	54%
5	Schulte 1996	97	10%	22%
6	Kavanagh 1993	69	16%	17%
7	1	2	3	4

4 COLUMNS

Fig. 8.3 Table for presentation. Seven rows and four columns limit is the basis for a table for presentation. Larger and complex tables have reduced readability

Only relevant data should find a place in such a table. Complex tables are ineffective; complex data may be given out in a printed handout. Tables from a journal or a book should not be photographed and used as a slide for presentation; such tables are difficult to read, have too many details for quick comprehension. A table that is spread out is more effective than a cluttered one; one should use the entire available screen area; however, this is not an invitation to increase entries in the table; larger space allows for use of larger fonts and bigger white spaces. Less is more; selection of appropriate information is important and effective. Vertical lines at the lateral borders of a table are omitted; almost all vertical lines in a table may be dropped for simplicity. One may use three horizontal lines: Two thick ones, between the table title and the column heading, and between the fields and the foot notes; one thin line between column heading and the data fields. One may sparingly use colour for emphasis. Too much colour in the background and in the text are annoying (Fig. 8.4).

Only the numbers that are needed to convince the audience of the results and conclusions may be used; rounding the presented values augments lucidity of tables (Fig. 8.5).

Text and data in a table must be accurate and consistent with the theme. Alignment of text and numbers in columns and rows is a prime property of an immaculate table; all the elements of a table—titles, headings, data, dividers, and notes should be well aligned. SI units are universally used in medical and scientific meetings (Fig. 8.6).

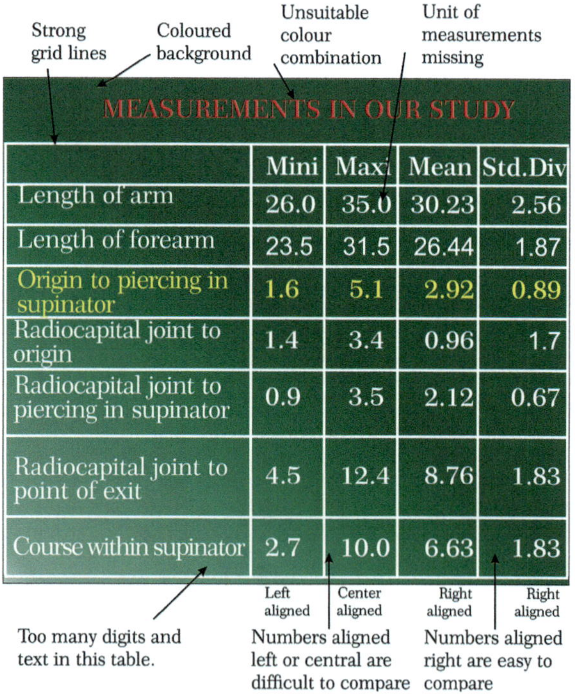

	Mini	Maxi	Mean	Std.Div
Length of arm	26.0	35.0	30.23	2.56
Length of forearm	23.5	31.5	26.44	1.87
Origin to piercing in supinator	1.6	5.1	2.92	0.89
Radiocapital joint to origin	1.4	3.4	0.96	1.7
Radiocapital joint to piercing in supinator	0.9	3.5	2.12	0.67
Radiocapital joint to point of exit	4.5	12.4	8.76	1.83
Course within supinator	2.7	10.0	6.63	1.83

Fig. 8.4 Table untenable. The values essential for the talk are highlighted in yellow; this is the only relevant measurement. The author had misused the table to summarize the entire data. Besides, there are other issues of readability. No one can blame the audience if they were disenchanted

State	Maharashtra	Karnatak	Goa
Population	81,538,628	58,491,643	4,106,586

A

State	Population
Maharashtra	81,538,628
Karnatak	58,491,643
Goa	4,106,586

B

State	Population
Maharashtra	81,538,628
Karnatak	58,491,643
Goa	4,106,586

C

State	Population (Millions)
Maharashtra	81.5
Karnatak	58.4
Goa	4.1

D

Fig. 8.5 Tables and numbers. Entering numbers in a table requires special attention. (**a**) It is tricky to compare numbers when they are placed in rows. The eyes have to look back-and-forth to compare one number to another. (**b**) It is easier to compare numbers when they are placed in a column, one below the other. In this example, the numbers are centre aligned to give a symmetrical appearance. Centre alignment creates confusion when one of the numbers has fewer digits. (**c**) The numbers in this column are right justified; this is the best arrangement to compare digits. (**d**) People often find it hard to deal with long numbers. Reducing digits and stating the value in millions or lakhs helps

How to design a presentational table

- Show only vital data; less is more
- Eschew templates; create a table
- Use maximal screen space; spread out the table
- Limit to 4 columns and 7 rows
- Minimum vertical and horizontal lines
- Enter title, column headings, row tags, and data
- Use large fonts
- Use colour to distinguish and not to decorate
- Use SI units, standard symbols and abbreviations
- Check correctness of text, numbers, and percentages

Fig. 8.6 Tenets of a presentational Table. A 10-point checklist to prepare a good table for presentation in a medical meeting

Figures

The term figure refers to any graphical display of measured quantities by means of the combined use of points, lines, a coordinate system, numbers, symbols, words, shading, or colour to create illustrative material used to present information or data [American Medical Association Manual of style 9E Williams & Wilkins 1998,

p. 66]. Figures include illustrations such as graphs, charts, algorithms, line drawing, computer generated images, and photographs. The purpose of a figure is to present information in a clear, concise, and accurate way. In scientific presentations graphs are used to showcase quantitative information. The frequently used graphs are discussed here. William Playfair (1759–1823) Scottish engineer and political economist is credited with inventing several types of figures like bar chart, line and area graphs, and pie chart. He is recognized as the founder of graphical methods of statistics.

Bar graph is a 1-axis graph and is used to compare amounts, frequencies, or magnitude of discontinuous data (Fig. 8.7). A bar graph may be vertical or horizontal. Vertical bar or column graph: One bar represents one category of data. Bars should have identical width and should be wider than the space between them. Bar length should be proportional to frequency. A figure may not have more than five to seven bars. The data is discrete, hence a baseline should not be drawn. Columns may be differentiated from each other by use of colours or shadings. Horizontal bar graph or chart is a variation; the horizontal orientation of the bars makes labelling easier. It is easier for people to read from left to right than from top to bottom; information placed from left to right is easier to follow. Requirements for horizontal display remain same as the vertical arrangement. Two or three columns may be put together in a grouped bar graphs; grouped bar graphs are unsuitable for presentation as it takes longer time to understand the information they represent. Deviation bar graph illustrates positive and negative information and is a good graphic to use.

Sub-divided (component) bar graph compares totals and proportions; each component is shown by a different colour. 100% bar graph compares components of a whole; most important data is near the baseline (Fig. 8.8).

Pie chart, its name comes from its resemblance to a pie. It has a circular shape and shows data in slices; group of data is represented by proportional slice of the pie. It is a simple and convenient figure to represent data visually as a fractional part of a whole (Fig. 8.9). Audience sees the data at a glance and understand the information quickly. This eliminates the need to examine underlying numbers themselves. A pie with up to 5 slices is easy to follow. The labels and numbers may be put outside and percentages inside the pie. A pie chart is good for one data set; comparisons of two pies is daunting task.

Data that can be shown in a pie chart can also be shown by another figure like component bar graph. It is easier to compare data in two component bar graphs than two pie charts. Pie does not easily show changes over time. If the number of slices goes over 7, then its readability suffers. Values are expressed in ratios or percentages which makes it difficult to know the exact value that is being represented. If one of the pies is less than 5%, then it should be pulled out, using the software, making it conspicuous. Presentation App has templates for 3D pies; these should be avoided; these do not add value, are tricky to follow and results are often mediocre. Doughnut chart is similar to a pie chart. Pie and doughnut charts may be used for talks for lay public but should be avoided in scientific presentations.

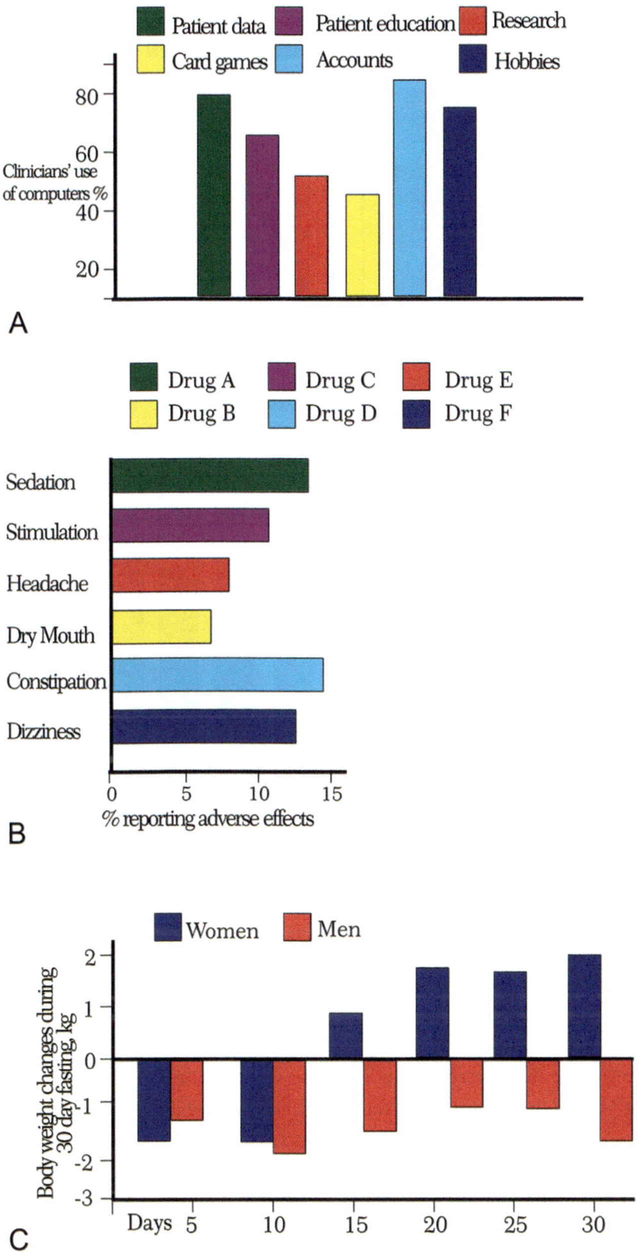

Fig. 8.7 Bars for presenting data (**a**) Column or vertical bar graph. Colours are used to differentiate between the 6 applications (**b**) Horizontal bar chart. Colours distinguish the reported side effects (**c**) Deviation bar graph. Horizontal rule at 0, shows no weight change, and is the baseline from which to compare weight loss or gain during fasting. Description of the axes in print media is always made parallel to their lengths; however, for reading convenience in a presentation a label for Y-axis may be set horizontally

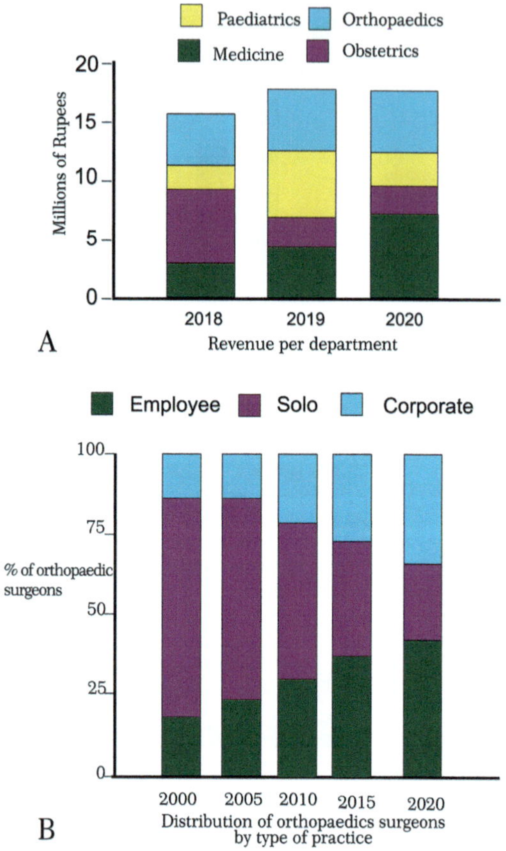

Fig. 8.8 Bars for presenting data (**a**) Component bar graphs. Different colours are used to represent components. Plots of values over time allow for comparison of trends of revenue of various departments (**b**) 100% bar graph. Comparative distribution of variables over time is shown. Variable of greatest interest is plotted nearest to the horizontal axis

Pictogram

Pictogram is a simple way of information presentation by placing a relevant picture with data. Picture of a car and bus to show their numbers in a city for example. A pictogram can also be used to display the components of a complex system or process and to demonstrate interrelations of these components.

Choropleth Map is one that uses differences in colouring and shading or placing symbols within specified areas to indicate the average values of a particular quantity in those areas. This is used to display trends or relationships that involve location and distance. For example, spread of a disease and its geographic locations are displayed in a map.

Histogram is a 2-axis graph that shows a frequency distribution by use of a series of contiguous rectangles (Fig. 8.10). The rectangles in a histogram should be of equal width and the location of the rectangle along the x-axis corresponding with the location of the interval within the group. The height and area of the rectangle corresponds to the frequency within the group. Frequency polygon is created by joining the data points with a line to show 2 or more frequency distributions. Midpoint of the frequency of each data class is selected.

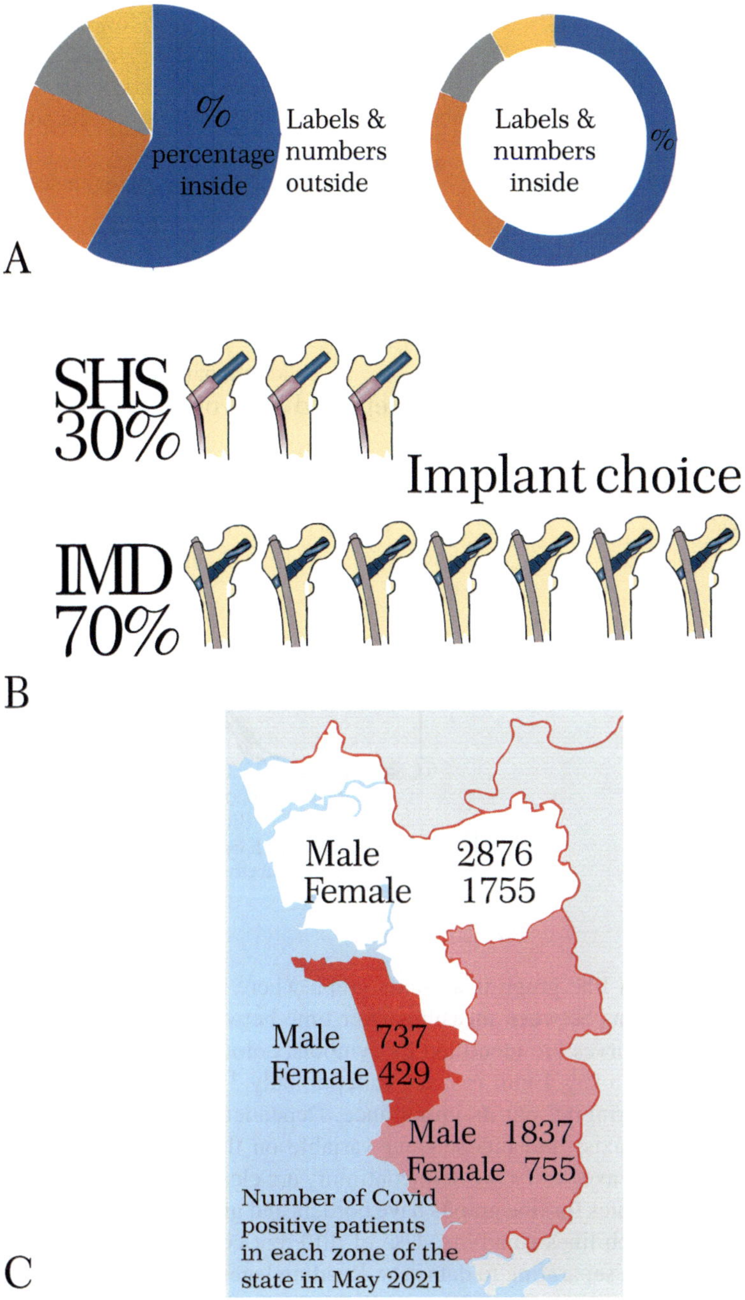

Fig. 8.9 Graphics in data presentation. (**a**) Pie chart is easy to understand and presents the data in a flash (**b**) Pictogram expresses the data with help of images of the concerned variables. (**c**) Choropleth map puts the data in perspective to geographic locations

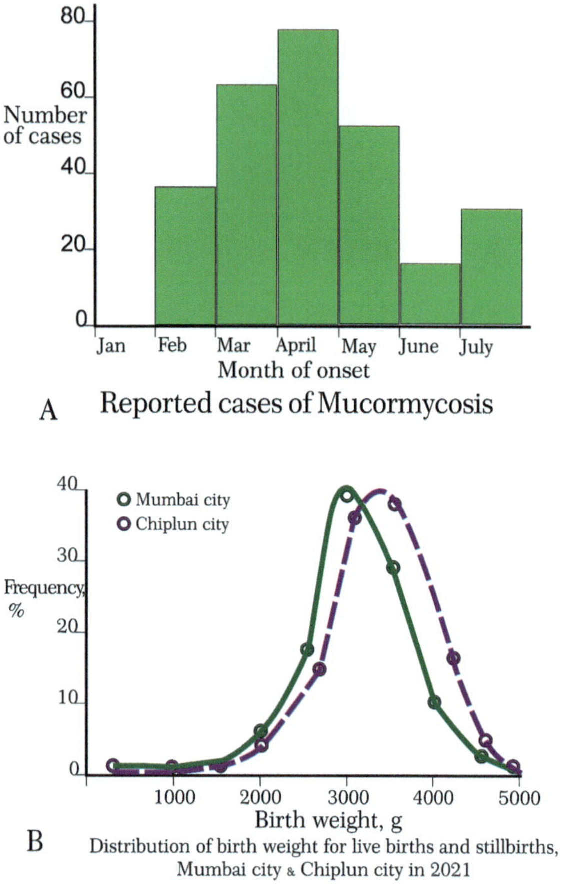

Fig. 8.10 Histogram and frequency polygon. (**a**) Histogram; relative frequency of infection in each month is shown. Height represents the number of cases for each month; width remains the same for all the columns. (**b**) Frequency polygon showing overlapping data on childbirth in two Indian cities. Horizontal positioning of a Y-axis label is convenient to read in a presentation, however, purist in the audience would expect it to be displayed parallel to its length i.e., vertical alignment

Line graph: A line graph is a 2-axis graph where data points or curves show changing relations between measures over time between 2 or more quantitative variables. The curves are identified by symbols, colours, or line width and these are explained in a key. Limit is 2 and exceptionally 3 curves. Animation of third curve helps in bringing out its importance. Dependent variable is shown on the vertical axis (y-axis) and independent variable on the horizontal axis (x-axis). Zero point of the axes and a break in continuity are clearly marked; adopt a simple scale. The templates for line graphs have borders and grids. These may be removed to make the graph lines stand out. Use of different colours and line thickness is more effective in separating to data sets. Reading legends in a projected chart and then following the lines is a difficult task for the audience; the graph lines when labelled should be easy to follow. With this display, the audience does not have to search the information as it is close to the lines and easy to find. The lines should have a name, a number, and text label in the same colour. A modification of line graph is area graph. The area between the axis and the line are highlighted with colours. These charts help to represent collected totals using numbers or percentages over time (Fig. 8.11).

Scattergram is a 2-axis graph with individual data points that show whether the data fit a mathematical function. If the dots cluster along a straight line, it shows evidence of linear relationship. When a relationship exists between independent (x-axis) and dependent (y-axis) the regression line through the data points shows the correlation. If the dots fall on a diagonal line, then the coefficient of correlation is 1.00. If there is no cluster, then there is no relationship.

Flow chart is useful to show flow patterns, sum-up complicated descriptions, study protocols and interventions (Fig. 8.12). Organizational charts show positions of individuals of a group (Video 8.1).

Decision tree is used in a decision analysis and evolves from left to right. Decision node is conventionally shown by a square. A chance node is shown by a circle and end node by a triangle. It is like a flow chart. Chance node is a point where a decision is made and ends in a decision. It has only burst nodes—splitting paths, but no sink nodes—converging paths. This chart grows like a big tree. It is well suited for progressive disclosure approach in a presentation (Fig. 8.13).

People remember pictures effortlessly in comparison to a text message. Length of a line, distance between two objects, relative height of two objects in 2D plain are easily identified. It is difficult to judge relative width of two objects, distance on a

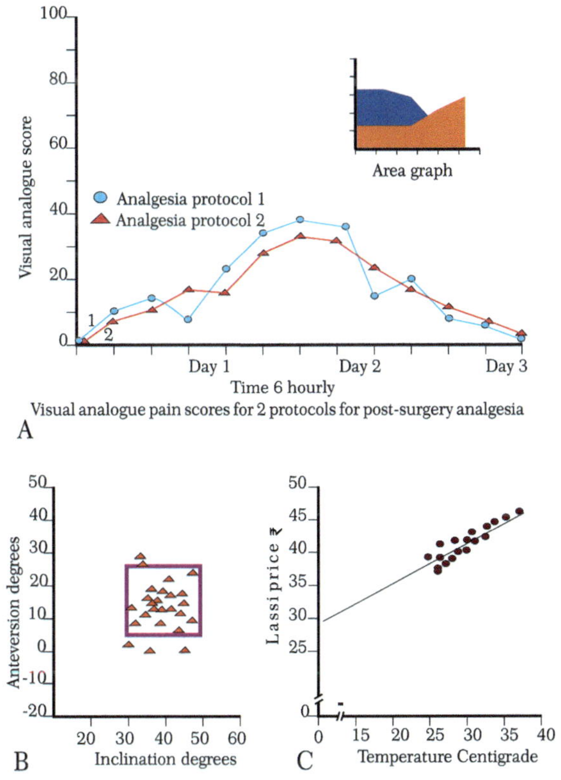

Fig. 8.11 Line and scatter graphs. (**a**) Line graph. The dependent variable is shown on the vertical axis—the Y-axis, and the independent variable is plotted on the horizontal axis—the X-axis. The symbols are explained in the figure key. Inset. area graph (**b**) Scatter graph showing angle and inclination of reconstructed acetabulae in total hip arthroplasty; a large number are within the safe zone (cluster) (**c**) Dots on a diagonal line represent correlation in this scatter graph; it suggests that the price of lassi grows in summer as the temperature increases

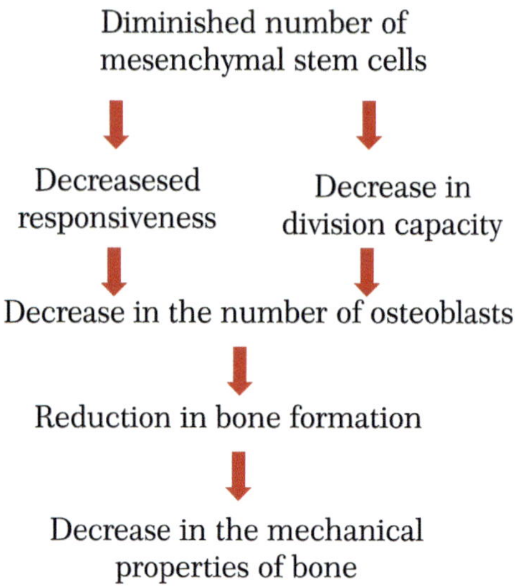

Fig. 8.12 Flow chart. Progress of a process is shown using top-to-bottom arrangement; arrows showing the sequence of events

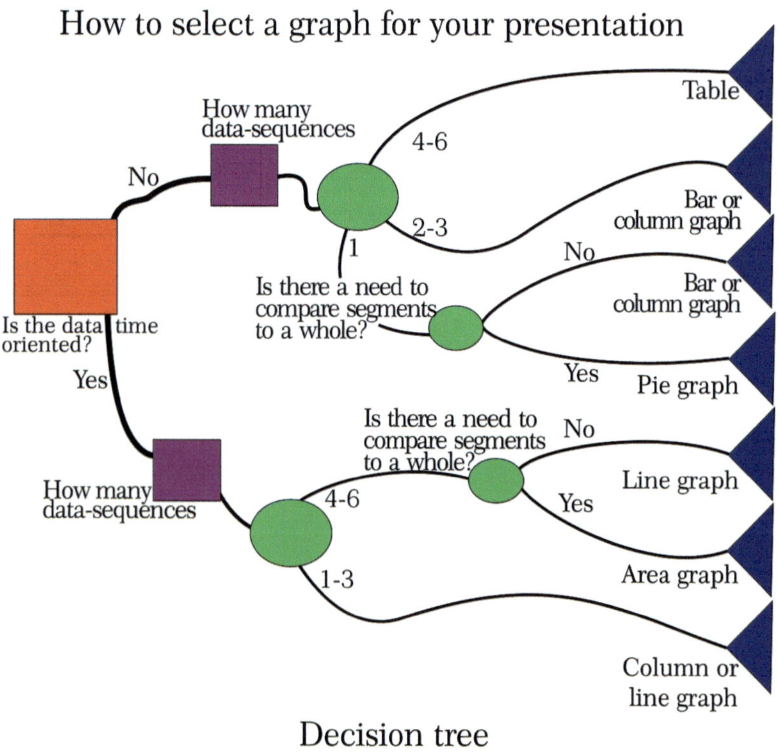

Fig. 8.13 Decision tree. Flow chart like diagram, a decision tree is simple to understand and interpret, needs minimum explanation

curved line, angle between two lines, and area of an object. Bodies shown in 3D dimension are hardest to judge and are often incorrectly estimated. This information is useful for selecting graphics for a presentation. Bar charts, line graphs, and dot scatter graphs are easily understood. Pie charts and area graphs are harder to appreciate and should be used with caution. 3D effect on any of the graphic, easily available on the computer and tempting to use for an impact is most confusing and should be avoided (Fig. 8.14). In a 2-axis chart the labels should be along the axis;

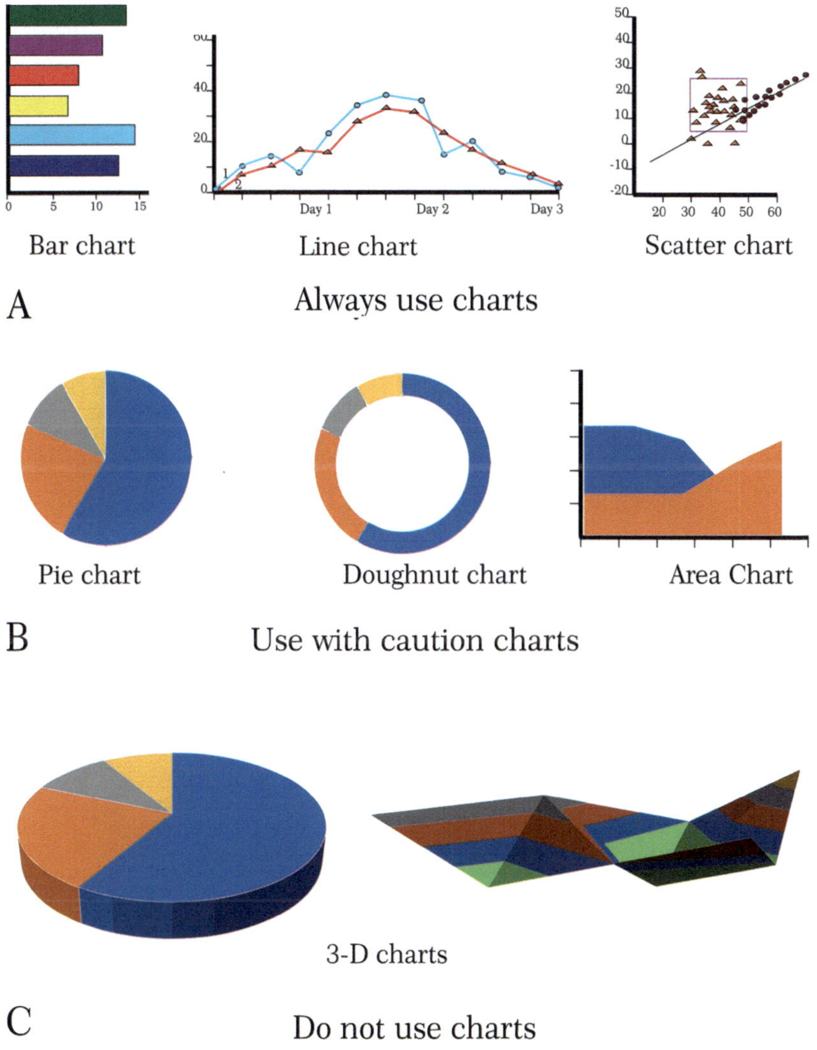

Fig. 8.14 Recommendations on use of graphics. (**a**) Charts that are easy to understand and may be used frequently (**b**) Charts that are difficult to follow and may be used with caution. (**c**) Charts that are confusing and at times misleading; should be avoided in medical presentations

Y-axis label is often difficult to read. If the audience is not hardcore professorial, then one may label the Y-axis horizontally. However, there is a risk of being labelled as unscientific presenter by a few in the audience.

A genealogy chart is a diagram that displays the frequency and development of phenotypes from one generation to the next of a single gene or organism and its descendants. These charts are prepared by using standardized designs and symbols (Fig. 8.15). In one presentation, the symbols should be consistent in a size. Generations are identified with roman numeral while individuals are indicated with hindu-arabic numeral placed in a consistent location, e.g. I-1, I-2, II-1. A male is represented by a square or symbol, a female is represented by a circle or symbol. Female partners are to the right of male partners. Siblings are drawn from oldest on the left to youngest on the right. These charts are ideal to record and display knowledge about a disease in a readable table and help in counselling the affected families.

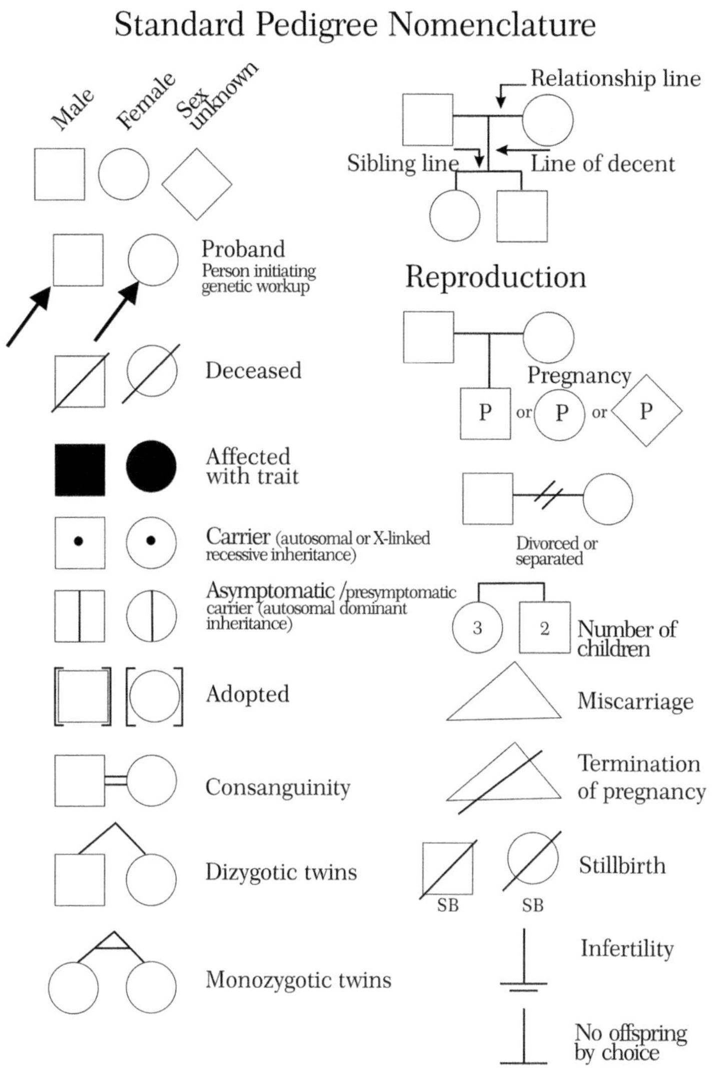

Fig. 8.15 Genealogy symbols. Standardized genealogical symbols support in precise communication of inherited conditions

Use of Photographs in Medical Presentations

9

'A picture is worth a thousand words'. – Arthur Brisbane 1911

Contents

Acquisition of clinical photographs is a topic for a separate book; some of its noteworthy aspects are mentioned here. Digital cameras are everywhere and general quality of digital picture is matching the images recorded on a film. Almost everyone involved in healthcare is now capable of taking a digital picture. This situation raises concern about patient's privacy.

Consent

Patient's informed consent is necessary before making preparations to photograph. The patient should be appraised not only of the purpose of recording the image but also who will see it, will it be copied, and distributed; will doctors, professional medical educators use it or a lay person may use it; how will it be secured and for how long (Fig. 9.1). The patient should be told beforehand whether an image is to be used for a book, or an article in a journal, or to be displayed on Internet or in an advertisement. Consent given by a patient who is under distress should be handled with extra care. If there are other persons in the photo, then their consent is necessary. Relatives may give consent only for a minor and not for an adult. It is safer to ask a third party to take the consent. Recording of a video or a photo must not delay

A. J. Thakur, *Tapping the Power of PowerPoint for Medical Posters and Presentations*, https://doi.org/10.1007/978-981-19-1816-2_9

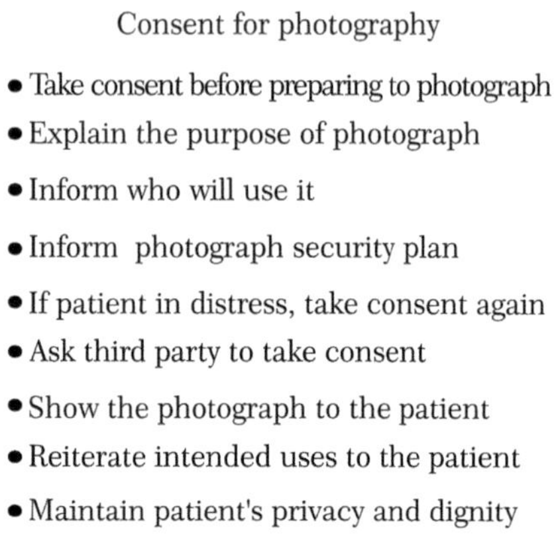

Fig. 9.1 Importance of patient's consent. Essential objectives enumerated

the treatment. It is prudent to show the recording to the patient and ensure that he or she is happy about the intended uses. In brief, it is wise to seek patient's permission without undue pressure to record and use an image and to give adequate information about its usage to all concerned. Stop the recording if the patient objects; do not participate in a recording against patient's wishes. Maintain patient's privacy and dignity. Use the digital recording only for purposes consented and keep it in secure conditions at all times. Formal written consent is not necessary to use images from pathology slides, roentgenograms, MRI, CT scans, ultrasound images, laparoscopic and arthroscopic images, and images of internal organs; verbal consent is adequate for these images.

Composition

The advantage of digital imaging is taking as many images as one wants and keeping the best ones. Composition is the arrangement of all the items that make up the theme of a photograph. The basic guidelines for composing a picture should be followed to get a quality image. The rule of thirds helps to place the subject in an optimum position. In photography, the rule of thirds of composition requires an image to be divided evenly into thirds, both horizontally and vertically, and the subject of the image be placed at the intersection of those dividing lines, or along one of the lines itself. Composition of a picture cannot be altered by image editing software.

In medical photography an uncluttered background makes a subject more noticeable. Wall posters, additional personnel, equipment, furniture, and fixtures are often seen in the background and these should be consciously avoided. The background can also be improved by treating the image in a photo editor but one needs to explicitly minimize background clutter. A clinician should create a permanent location with a plain background to shoot good quality clinical photographs. In general, one should take a series of images at varying distances and angles and choose the suitable ones for presentation.

Lighting

Photographs should be taken in ambient light. Use of flash is complex because it is difficult to control the strong shadows cast by its bright light. When comparable images are needed, these may be created by using the same lighting, patient position, camera zoom level, and distance from the subject, e.g. If a flash is used for 'before' picture, it must be used for 'after' image as well. Good closeup images require meticulous focusing.

Regional Photography

Photographing an oral cavity requires special lenses and lighting (Fig. 9.2). In dental photography the cosmetic standard series include 17 views which are required twice, before and after the treatment. Digital photography is a boon for dental imaging as the cost of a single image is minimal after the equipment has been installed. Patient's consent becomes critical as it is easier to identify a person in dental photographs than other parts of the body.

It is tricky to photograph skin lesions; tone should be close to reality and lesions in sharp focus. Natural ambient lighting is optimal for skin photos. The target area should be placed on a firm support. If the lesion is on torso, patient should lie down.

Head and neck photographs come out best against a matt finish white background. Black or dark blue colours also make a good background. Yellow and red colours dominate the image and may not be used. A horizontal line drawn from the external auditory canal to the infra-orbital rim is known as the Frankfort plane. It is a useful guide to photograph head and neck. When the line is horizontal, the face is forward looking without an up or down tilt.

Ophthalmic photographs are of numerous types: fundus imaging, angiography, OCT (Optical Coherence Tomography) imaging, slit lamp imaging, external photography to name a few. Specialized lenses and cameras are required for quality pictures. Patient consent is important when using external eye photos for presentation.

Endoscopic images are regularly obtained during the course of the work. Digital format has made it easy to store these in large quantities. These endoscopic images can be used in teaching, conference, research, and publication. Furthermore, if any medicolegal issues arise, this good practice protects both the endoscopist and the patient. Verbal consent is adequate to use endoscopic images for presentation.

Photography in the operating room is tricky. The operating lights are unsuitable for photography because they are very bright and cause apparent total darkness at the image periphery. Ring flash is a useful device for photographing cavities. Standard flash works sub minimally; it is safer to photograph in ambient light. Use of a tripod is recommended when slower exposures are required; this avoids blurred images. Orientation in an intra-operative photograph could be problematic. Additional images of a body landmark like neck or hand are useful to establish a

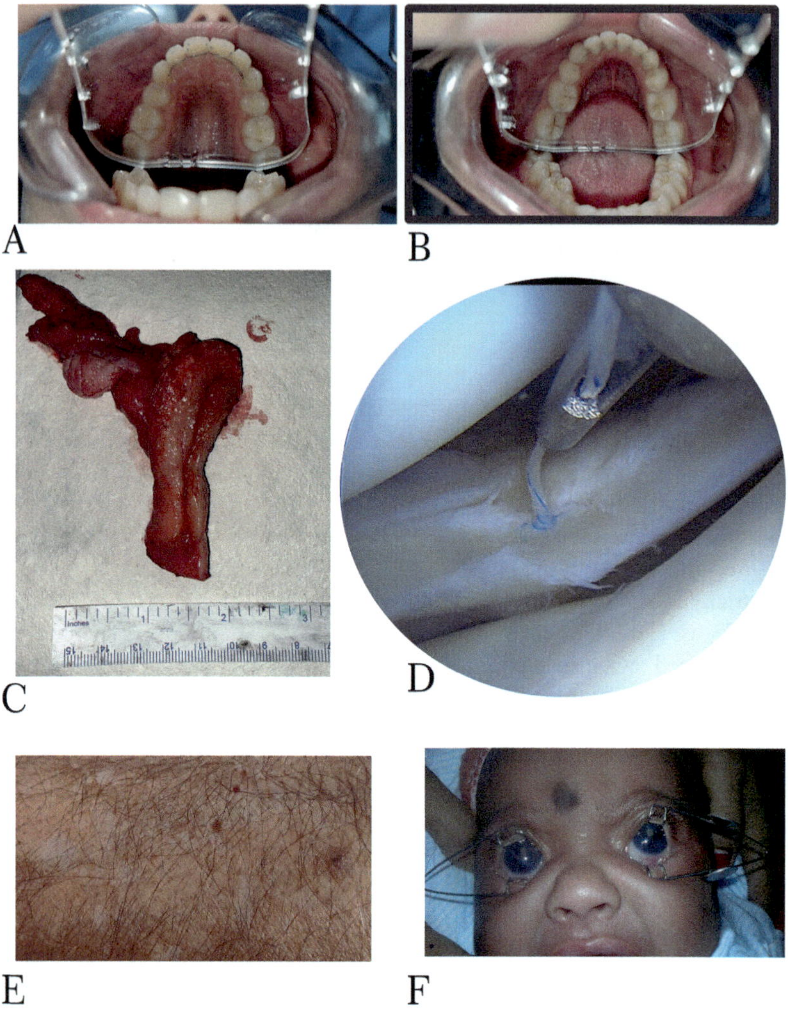

Fig. 9.2 Clinical photographs. (**a**) Special lens and ring flash are used to photograph oral cavity. (**b**) Placing a square border sets apart the photograph and improves the detail of the picture (**c**) Inclusion of a ruler is useful when photographing a surgical specimen. (**d**) Endoscopic (arthroscopic) photograph of meniscus repair in the knee joint. (**e**) A lesion photographed in natural ambient light shows skin colour close to reality. (**f**) Ophthalmic patients require a wide range of clinical imaging

perspective; keeping the same orientation photographs of the area of interest may be taken.

Intra-operative photographs should be shot from the surgeon's eye view; avoid shooting over-the-shoulder views. The surgeon should stand aside when photographs are taken. It may be necessary to stand on a stepladder or a stool and record images from above; the camera should be directly above the wound. The photographer must be guided to target the area of interest; several images with minor variation may be taken and the best one may be used for presentation, a convenience in the digital age.

The surgical wound should be cleaned up before a shot; blood wiped away from the area. A short saline wash and wiping the area makes it cleaner and presentable. A change of soiled green or blue drapes makes a good picture. All unused instruments may be removed from the area. Retractors may remain but reflections off the metal should be controlled. New or clean gloves for the person holding the retractor is a smart move. Cautery wire and suction tube should be out of the picture zone. Circulating OT personnel may be asked to hold a drape to arrange a neutral background. To create a sense of proportion, a scale may be placed in the surgical field; a floppy ruler that comes with a sterile marking pen is a handy choice; metal rulers reflect light. If a series of photos are being taken for sequential disclosure of a procedure, then all the photographs should be taken from the same spot, with the same camera, lens settings, and same illumination.

The surgical specimen should be placed flat on a firm, clean white surface in abundant ambient light. The camera should be parallel to it and be placed directly above it, on a tripod if possible. Whenever a specimen is photographed, a ruler should be included in the view (see Fig. 9.2). This eliminates the need to explain the magnification.

All original image files should be saved separately and securely. A copy of the file should be used for processing for presentation.

Image Editors

Image editing programs are specialized software for image enhancement. They help to elevate and perfect a photograph by achieving correct exposure, colouration, focus, contrast, and brightness. Editing programs also help in cropping and magnifying an image; in removal and change of shape of existing objects, or even introduce new objects in an image. It is feasible to create a medical image with completely fabricated abnormalities and it is difficult to detect such duplicity.

A speaker should not distort the truth by modifying photographs using computer skills. Electronic modification of photos should be limited to cropping, sizing, colour correction, minor tonal enhancement, clean-up of dust spots or scratches. These changes should be done responsibly and should not be used to alter scientific contents; coverup and distortion of clinical photographs constitute scientific fraud. Journal editors expect to see original and modified medical images before a paper is published. In medical meetings the organizers do not exert such a control but expect the speakers to present their material with integrity; the scientific honesty of academic presentations is maintained largely by the honour system among researchers. There is no place for trickery in presenting scientific results.

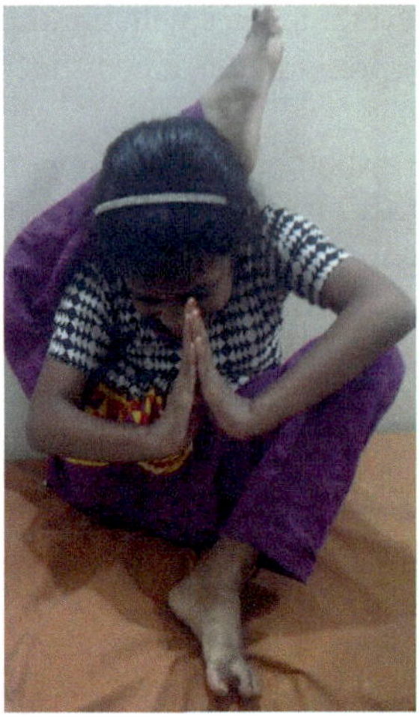

A

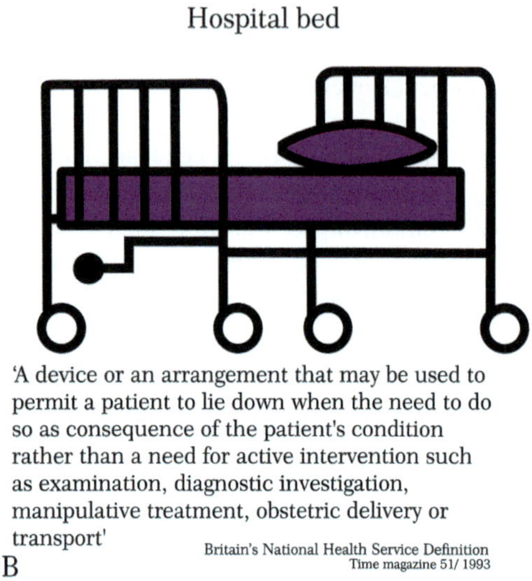

B

Fig. 9.3 (**a**) It is easier to show a picture than to describe this 'aasan' in words, (**b**) A hospital bed—a sketch and in words

How to show a Photograph

Photographs play a major role in a medical presentation for various reasons. It saves lots of spoken words needed to describe a complex situation; it is simpler to show a picture than to describe this 'aasan' (Fig. 9.3). Leonardo da Vinci said, 'do not bother with words, show them a picture'.

Photography is the perfect medium to show a scientific object or a clinical condition. A photograph should be adequately labelled for quick understanding. It is quite common to see a photo-montage in a presentation; speakers often want to show all the information in one slide (Fig. 9.4).

Audience can grasp only one picture at a time. If one shows 6 steps at a go, it becomes difficult to comprehend all the steps in that short time a slide is on the screen; the speaker feels he has shown a lot, the audience gains little. ['The single biggest problem in communication is the illusion that it has taken place'.—George Bernard Shaw.] It is better to break down such a slide in smaller units; each unit may be enlarged and put up as an individual slide, each slide can be adequately labelled and described as it is being shown. The audience needs guidance and the easiest way is to insert a line sketch of the objects seen in an intra-operative photograph (Fig. 9.5). Intra-operative photographs should be shown with extra effort; a speaker is always well versed with an intra-operative photograph and can identify all the minute details because he has seen it several times. Audience who sees it for the first time and needs to be explained the details with line sketches, labelling, computer generated block arrows suitably animated and narration.

Photographs of before and after sequences are very useful in a presentation (Fig. 9.6).

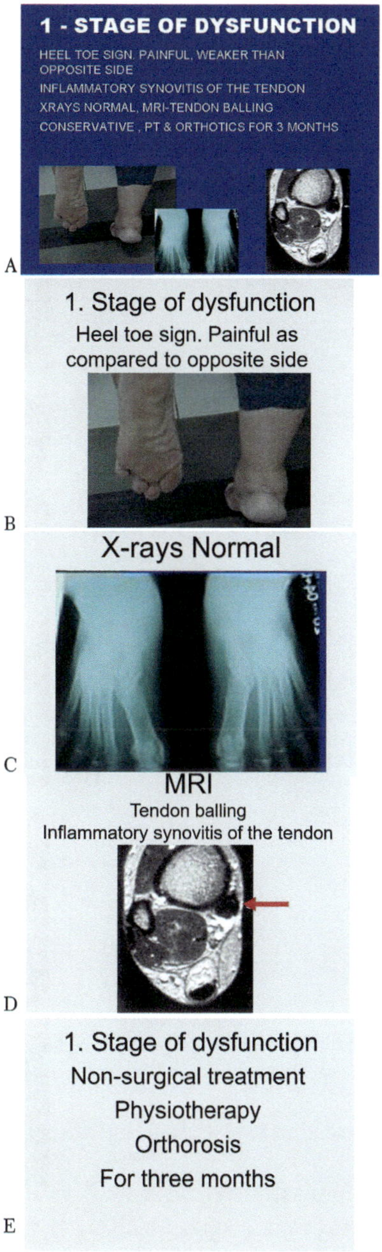

Fig. 9.4 Too many details. (**a**) Too much information is laid out in one slide; this is difficult to understand. The same material is distributed over 4 slides showing (**b**) clinical features, (**c**) X-ray, (**d**) MRI scan with an arrow, and (**e**) treatment, making matters simple for the audience. Time required to discuss slide a or other 4 is the same but lucidity improves

Only clear and crisp photographs are well seen on a big screen. In digital photography an image deteriorates on repeated resizing and saving. A picture that looks hazy on the computer screen looks worse when projected; all the imperfections are enlarged several times. Always use high-quality photographs for projection.

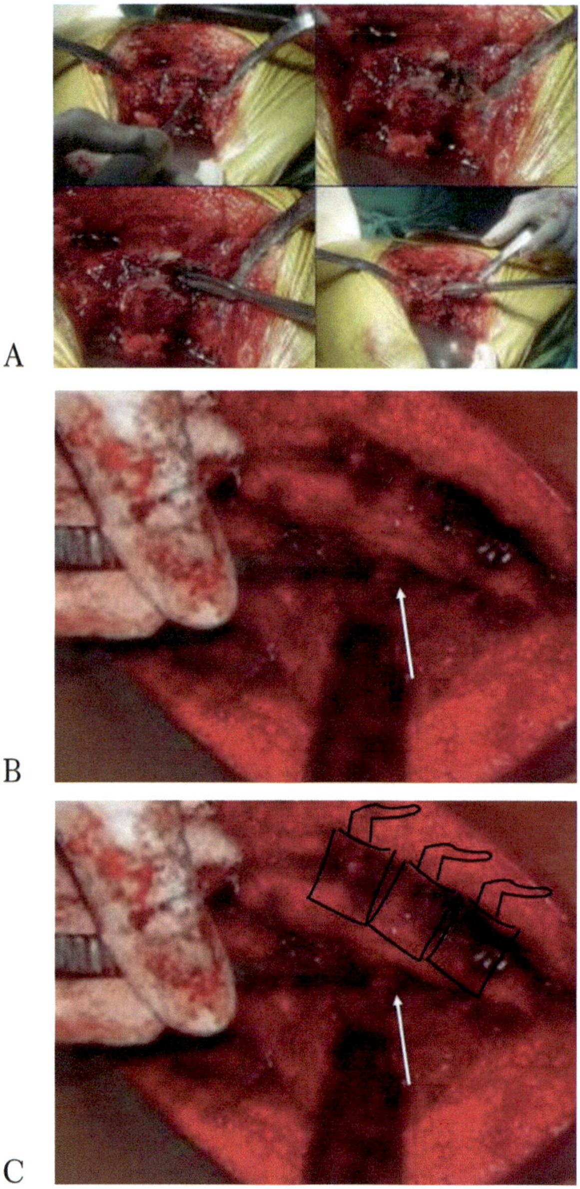

Fig. 9.5 Intra-operative photograph. (**a**) montage of 4 steps of a procedure leaves a vague impression. (**b**) Showing one of the pictures with an arrow makes it more useful (**c**) Superimposing a line sketch puts things in perspective

If a break in sequence of showing the slides is needed, then it is better to use a blank slide; a filler photograph is a distraction and may not be used. A photograph that relates to the message and makes it clear, may only be shown (Fig. 9.7).

Use the screen to the maximum. Slide layouts in presentation programs put a frame around a picture space. This leaves a lot of white (blank) space on the screen. This design is good for mounting a painting for exhibition. In a presentation aim is

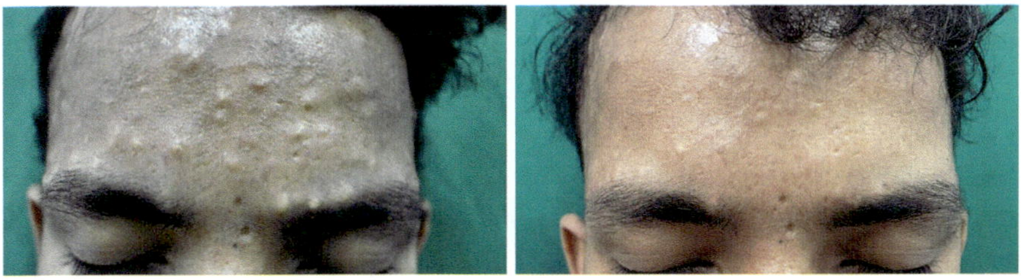

Before After

Fig. 9.6 Photographs showing regression of a lesion before and after the treatment

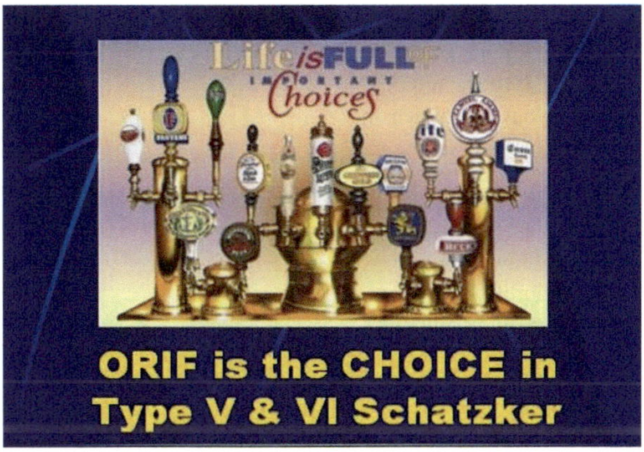

Fig. 9.7 Relevance of the image to the topic being discussed is farfetched, if at all

to show a picture in its maximum possible size on the screen so the audience can see all the details. If one uses the default layouts, the picture size is reduced which defeats the purpose of showing a picture. Largest possible picture should be shown on the screen (Fig. 9.8).

A picture should make an impact and not serve as a decoration on 'prompt card' slide (Fig. 9.9).

Microscopic pictures should always be shown with a scale; a ruler should be incorporated. Use of wooden or laser beam pointers should be minimal when showing a microscopic image; use of computer arrows to indicate areas of interest is more efficient as it saves time and is precise (Fig. 9.10).

A photograph should be sharp, clear, and without distortion when shown on a screen, every time.

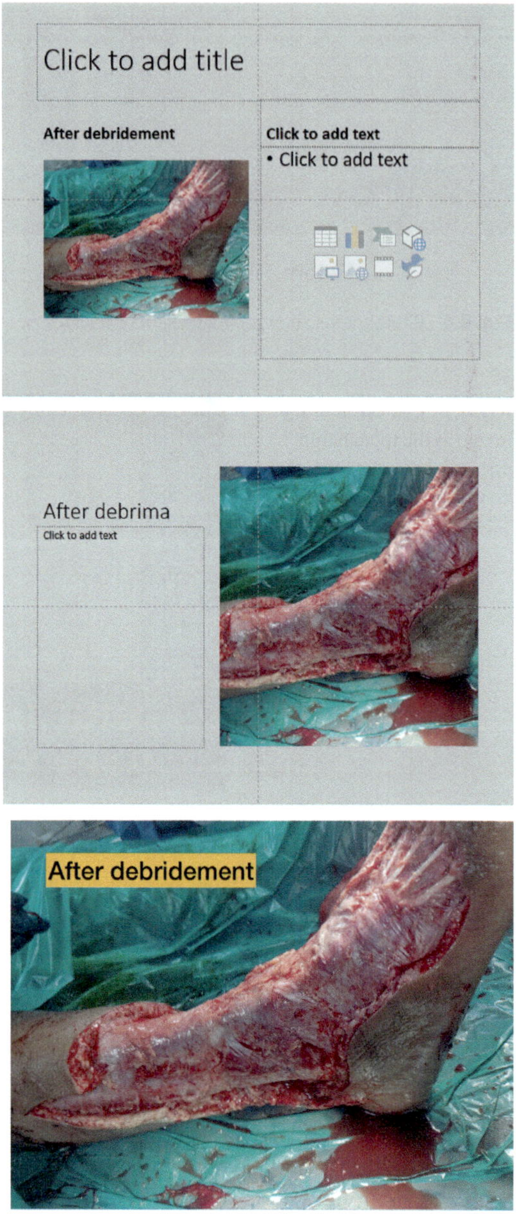

Fig. 9.8 Display largest image. Presentation programs offer insert boxes in the slides that automatically resize an image. However, the size of the image is reduced as seen in (**a** and **b**) There is a lot of blank space around the image which now resembles a mounted picture in a frame; this is a good arrangement from artistic point of view to display a picture but greatly reduces its size; a medical photograph requires clarity and not artistic layouts. (**c**) When an image is inserted on a blank slide, it can be resized to occupy the available space, enhancing clarity and improving image legibility; if required, it can be suitably labelled

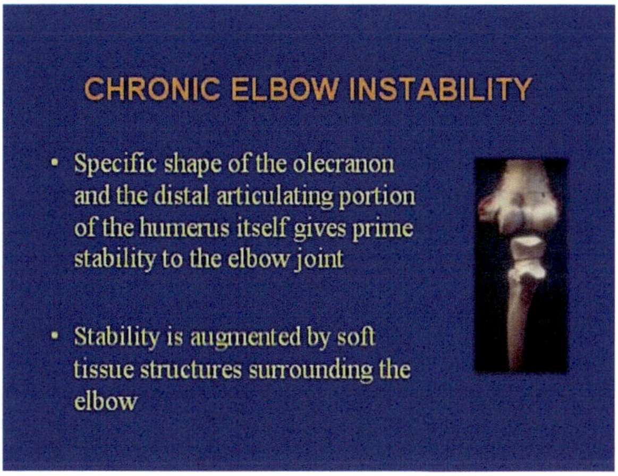

Fig. 9.9 The picture is indeed related to subject but makes little impact because of poor details and inadequate labelling, ends up just as a decoration on a prompt card slide

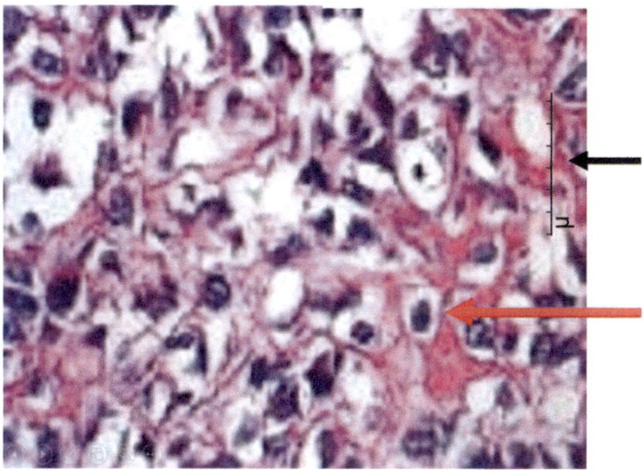

Fig. 9.10 Showing a microscopic slide. A ruler should be included (black arrow). Use of a computer generated arrow (red arrow) is recommended for accuracy and time saving

Showing X-Ray, MRI, CT, and Ultrasound Images in Presentations

10

Contents

History of X-Rays

Ever since the discovery in 1895 by Wilhelm Roentgen, X-rays prints are being displayed in medical meetings. Roentgen himself showed an X-ray of his wife's hand at several meetings. X-ray prints were commonplace by 1912 as celebrated British orthopaedic surgeon Robert Jones observed, 'Patients who call upon me are often armed with X-ray prints, which they authoritatively expound. Anything but a faultless end to end apposition imparts a war-like spirit'; one hundred and ten years later, things are almost similar. Presently X-ray images are ubiquitous in all clinical meetings, more so in orthopaedics, dentistry, and radiology.

X-Ray Image Acquisition

Acquiring X-ray images for presentation requires efforts. A SLR camera should be used for better images. The camera may be mounted on a tripod; this avoids minor

Supplementary Information The online version contains supplementary material available at [https://doi.org/10.1007/978-981-19-1816-2_10].

A. J. Thakur, *Tapping the Power of PowerPoint for Medical Posters and Presentations*, https://doi.org/10.1007/978-981-19-1816-2_10

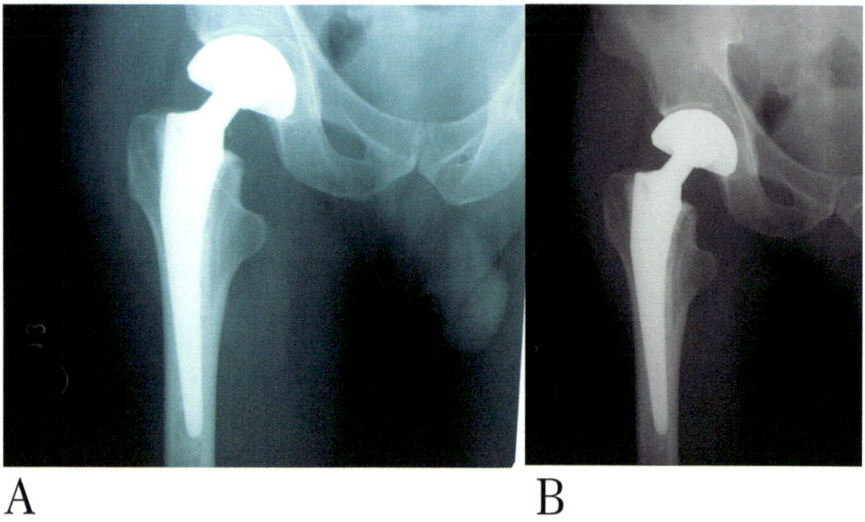

Fig. 10.1 Blue tinge x-ray. (**a**) Photographed X-ray often attains an unnatural blue tinge when copied on a viewing box. (**b**) Such an image should be processed to grayscale in an image editing software. All available space on a slide should be used to display an X-ray

shakes and helps in sharp focusing on areas of interest. When needed zoom should be used to narrow the field of vision. Digital cameras offer option to shoot in black and white mode. X-rays should be photographed in this mode. If such an option is unavailable, the image should later be processed in a photo editing app to create a grayscale image. X-ray images with blue tinge appear unnatural and may not be used in presentations (Fig. 10.1).

X-ray film should be put up on an evenly lit viewing box; the lighting should be pushed to maximum; new LED viewing box is preferred over the conventional backlit one (Fig. 10.2). View box clips that hold the film in place make an inelegant picture. Eliminate these clips from being photographed; stick the X-ray film in middle of the viewing box with removable, reusable adhesive putty.

Use of phone camera is widespread in healthcare environment. Expensive phone camera does not guarantee high-quality copy of the X-ray film unless shot carefully. All the room lights are switched off to avoid reflection from the film or the view box surface. A phone camera held very close to the view box may record the reflection of the photographer superimposed on the X-ray film; an embarrassing situation that is tedious to correct in a Photoshop like apps. Holding the phone camera farther away and using zoom avoids this unpleasant situation. Unwanted light is minimized by covering the illuminated area around the X-ray film with a cardboard, whenever possible. The phone camera should be parallel to the film surface to avoid distortion. Camera flash should be switched off. All modern phone cameras come with filter technology; grayscale filter should be applied in the camera app before shooting to get natural looking grayscale copy of the X-ray film. An X-ray film may have AP/lateral/oblique views; copying each view separately ensures superior image details. Generous margin around the object of interest should be maintained while

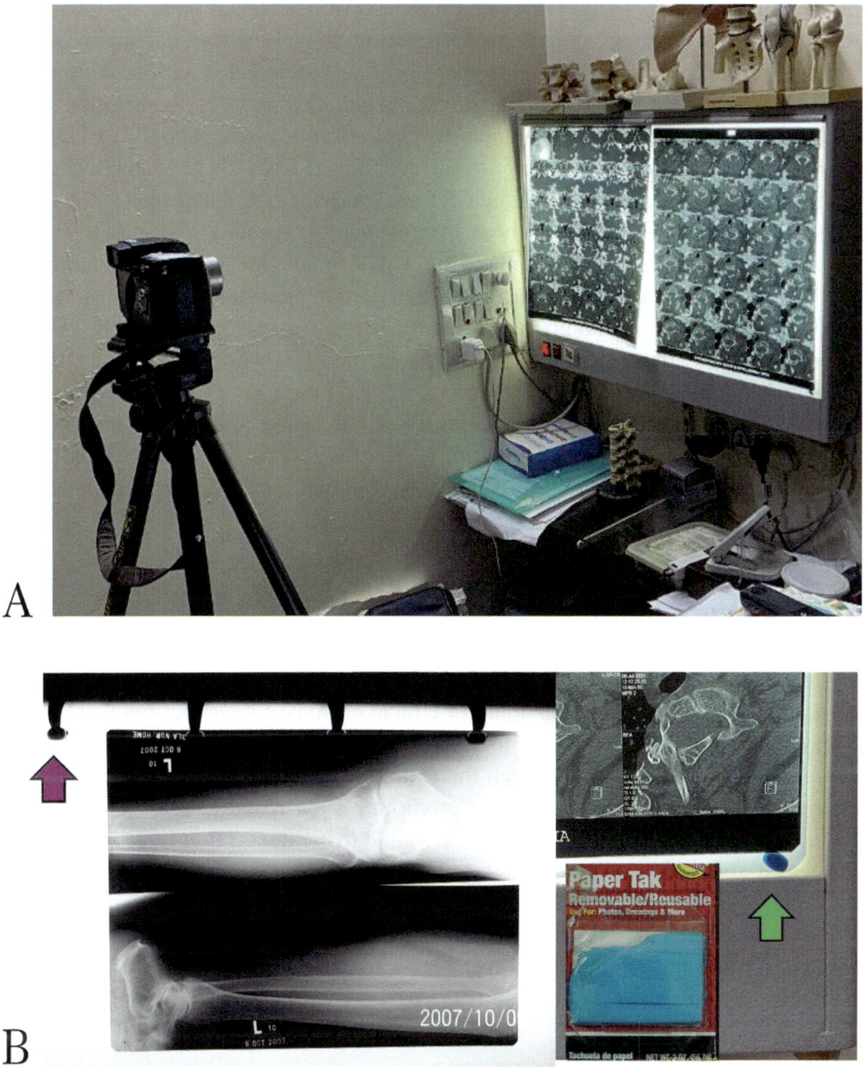

Fig. 10.2 Setup to acquire X-ray images for presentation. (**a**) SLR camera mounted on a tripod. This facilitates sharp focusing and eliminates shake. The camera is parallel to the film surface. (**b**) The film is placed on a backlit view box. Clips (magenta arrow) are not much to look at when projected. The film should be secured by reusable and removable putty (green arrow)

shooting.; margin may then be cropped as required; if the copy is distorted, perspective may be edited in a photo app.

Procurement from an X-ray workstation is easy and quality of image obtained is high. DICOM is the original language for all medical imaging. DICOM images can be exported to JPEG or BMP; for a DICOM image an exported JEPG file is smaller (e.g. 597 kb) than a BMP file (e.g. 3.59 MB). Both these formats, on projection look indistinguishable. These are grayscale images and are presentation ready. Quality of these images is superior to one copied by photography. Besides, such an image can carry patient's data; when exporting there is an option to get it with or without the data. One must hide patient identification data while using it for presentation.

Images procured by photographing the CRT (Cathode Ray Tube) or LED (Light Emitting Diode) screen are inferior to those obtained from image intensifier's hard disc. The horizontal lines seen on the CRT screen reduce the details and stand out as a sore thumb. A few years ago, those images were the best of what was available, but now they belong to the past. Image intensifier images are stored on its hard disc, can be copied to a portable storage device and used in presentations (Fig. 10.3). This mode of retrieval ensures high visual quality of the images.

MRI and CT images are usually given out on a CD where a copy of DICOM reader is preloaded and displays the images. Each image is of high quality and can be copied and pasted directly on a slide. When CD is unavailable then images may be photographed from the printed film. One needs to be selective in picking up important cut for display. Use of tripod mounted camera and zoom lens is useful. Sharp focus is necessary.

X-Ray Image Editing

Digital X-ray images can be easily manipulated with the available apps. Such manipulation is welcome when done for ethical reasons, e.g. an incorrectly exposed X-ray may be digitally corrected to visualize actual findings, remove artefacts and defects. It amounts to a fraud when the technology is used for wrong reasons like alter findings with ulterior motives or promoting a particular technology or a technique for commercial benefit. It is now possible to create X-ray images with totally fabricated abnormalities and such deceit is difficult to detect. Digital modification of X-rays should be done with discretion and never for change of scientific content. It should be restricted to tonal adjustments, cropping, sizing, clearing dust spots and scratches. If in a presentation an object has been removed to highlight certain aspect, it should be mentioned in the slide (Fig. 10.4). There is no place for chicanery in presenting medical matters.

X-Ray Presentation

Displaying X-rays in a presentation requires groundwork. A typical X-ray film has a lot of unused space and should be cropped to keep only the areas of interest (Fig. 10.5). Slides in the Presentation program have insert boxes which automatically resize an image, but leave a lot of space around it. The inserted X-ray then appears like a mounted painting. Reduced size of the X-ray translates to its decreased

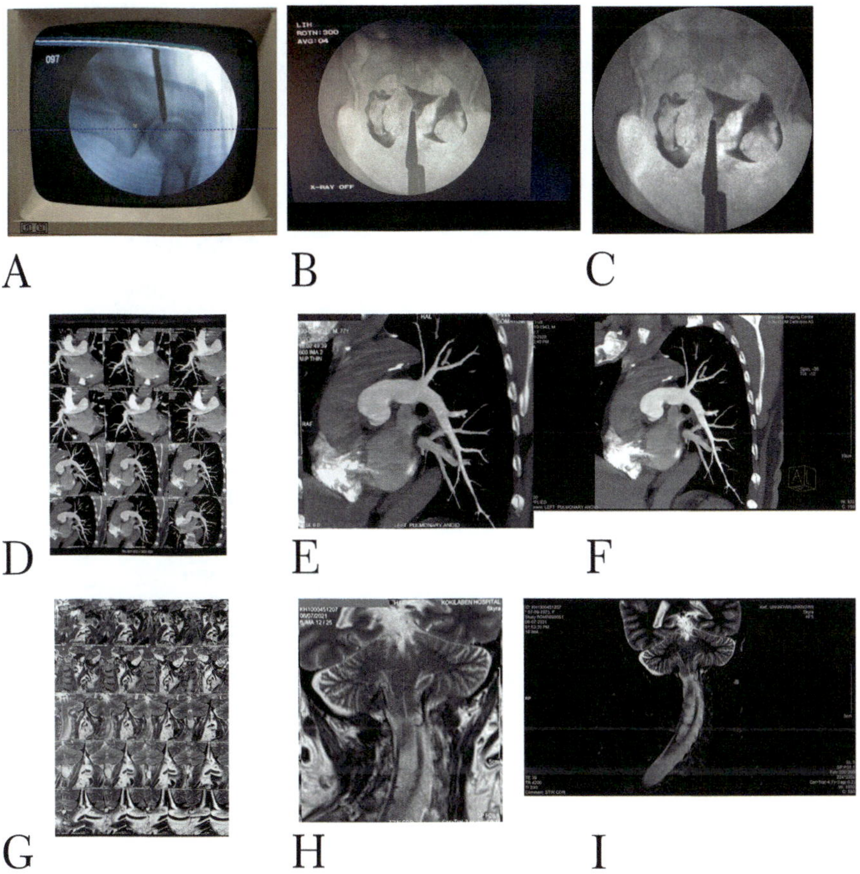

Fig. 10.3 Image acquisition from various sources. (**a**) CRT screen photographed. Horizontal lines across the screen reduce image sharpness. (**b**) LED screen photographed. (**c**) Copied from the image intensifier console; image has fine details in grayscale; projection ready. (**d**) Printed sheet of CT scan of chest photographed. Difficult to follow details on projection; difficult to conceal patient ID because each square carries full patient data. (**e**) One square from the sheet photographed. Shows objects in detail and patient identity can be concealed. (**f**) Same square copied from the CD; grayscale image with finer details. (**g**) Printed sheet of MRI scan of cervical spine photographed. (**h**) Closeup of a square and (**i**) copied from CD

legibility, a side effect of poor designing of the slide by the app programmer who has little understanding of the needs of the medical profession. The larger the X-ray image the better the legibility. In a slide, all available space should be used to display an X-ray. Progressive disclosure technique is useful in explaining a subtle point in an X-ray (Video 10.1).

Indispensable X-ray images some times are of poor quality but their clarity can be improved in an imaging app. Another way to achieve improved X-ray legibility is to highlight the contour of the object (Fig. 10.6). The topic under discussion can

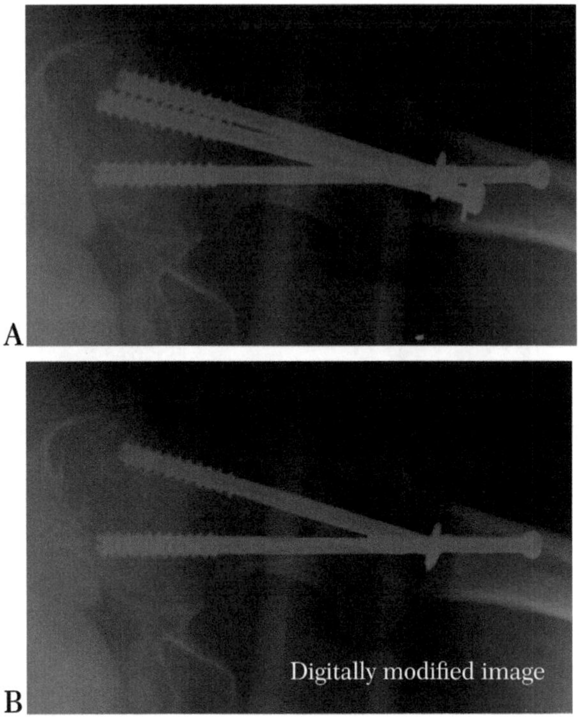

Fig. 10.4 Image alteration. (**a**) Original X-ray of fracture fixation. (**b**) One screw was digitally removed to emphasize a certain aspect of the technique. Though alteration was innocuous, a disclosure is essential

be explained better by showing a line drawing or a photograph together with an X-ray (Fig. 10.6b).

Montage

It is common to see a large number of X-rays displayed in a single slide to illustrate multiple aspects of problem, a concept, or a procedure (Fig. 10.7). The speaker believes showing different levels of a process at a glance, may explain the entire issue instantly. Audience has limited time to concentrate on an image, finds it difficult as small size of the image does not encourage concentration and shortly gives up on that slide. The collage technique is valuable in a print media or in a poster when several images can be studied at individual's convenience and speed. In a live meeting such photomontages are ineffective.

Never apologize for poor quality of an X-ray; just do not show one. Nothing is achieved by showing poor-quality X-rays; it is a waste of time and audience does not get the message (Fig. 10.8). It is better to use those thousand words to describe the object than showing a poor-quality X-ray.

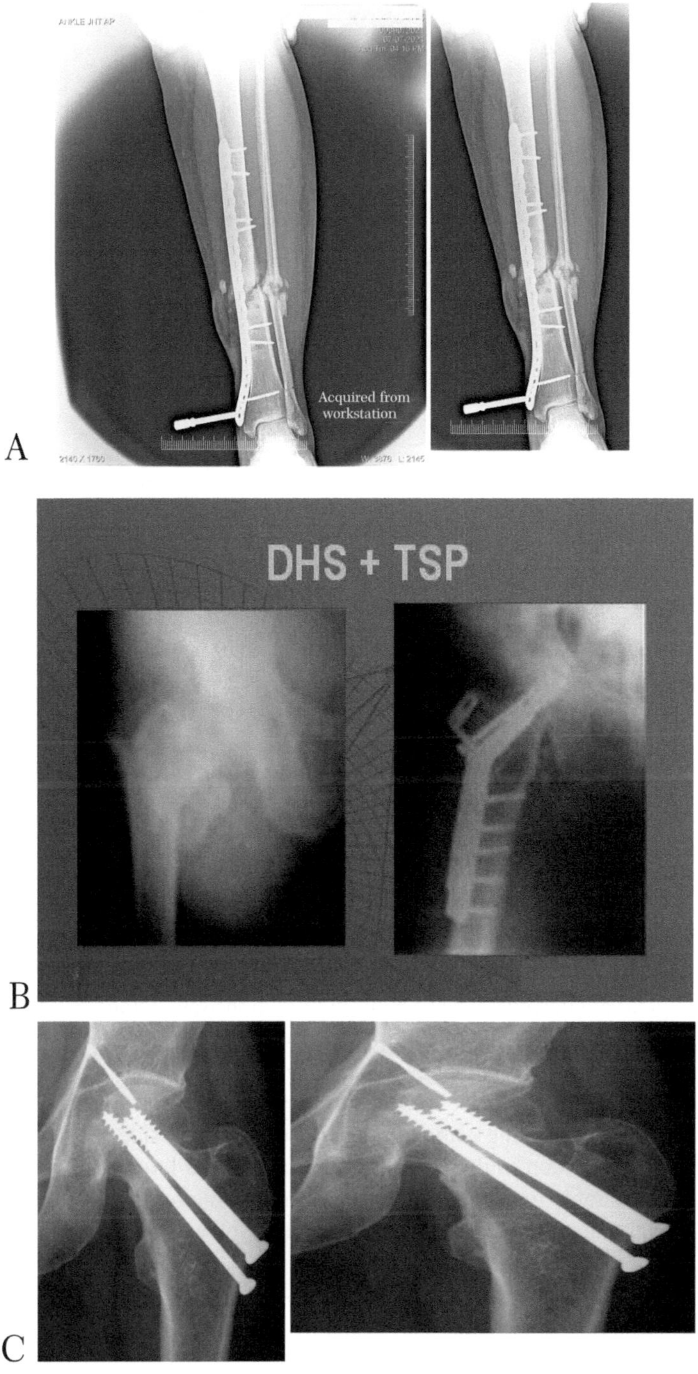

Fig. 10.5 Size reduction. (**a**) Crop out inessential area of a typical X-ray and retain the part of interest. (**b**) X-rays are reduced in size in insert box leaving considerable unused space on the slide. (**c**) An X-ray image should be proportionally enlarged. It distorts if stretched in one axis to fill up the slide

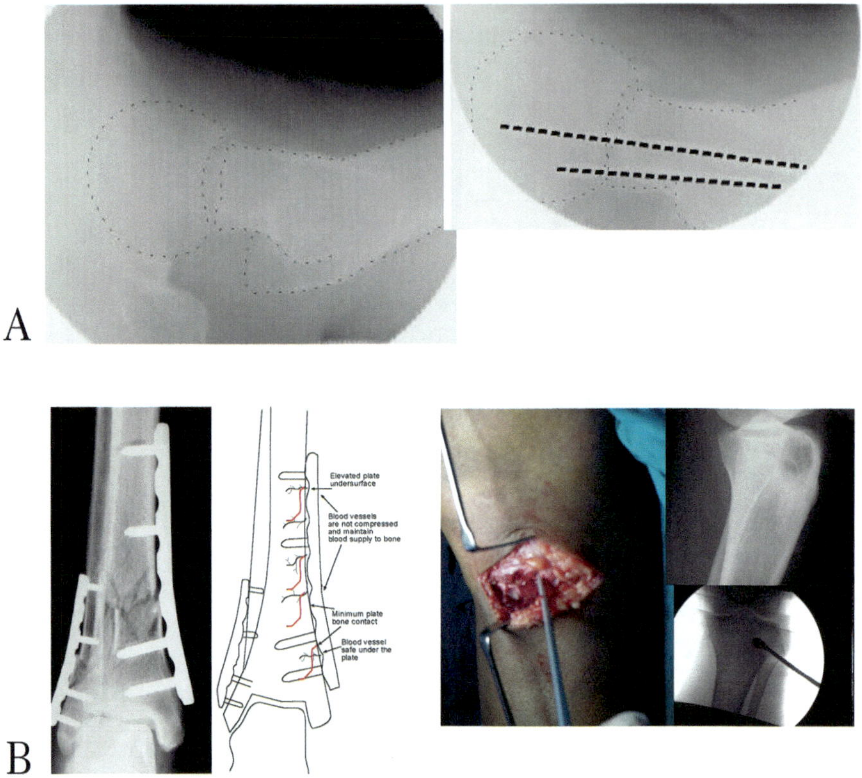

Fig. 10.6 Improving X-ray's legibility. (**a**) Highlighting faint outline of an object in a poor-quality X-ray image improves its readability. (**b**) Presenting an X-ray in combination with a line sketch or a photograph greatly increases its usefulness

Computer Generated Arrows

Computer generated arrows should be used to demonstrate details of an X-ray. Use of a laser beam pointer should be minimized or eliminated; it is a time waster; to use it one needs to pickup it up, spot the object on the big screen, aim with a steady hand and shoot, wait for the audience to concentrate before you speak, all this takes time which can be saved by using computer generated arrows. Besides, laser beam pointers are ineffective when multiple screens are in use in a large conference. Mouse pointer is comparable to a laser pointer in terms of time requirement and does not score over automated block arrows. Pre-conference planning is necessary for using

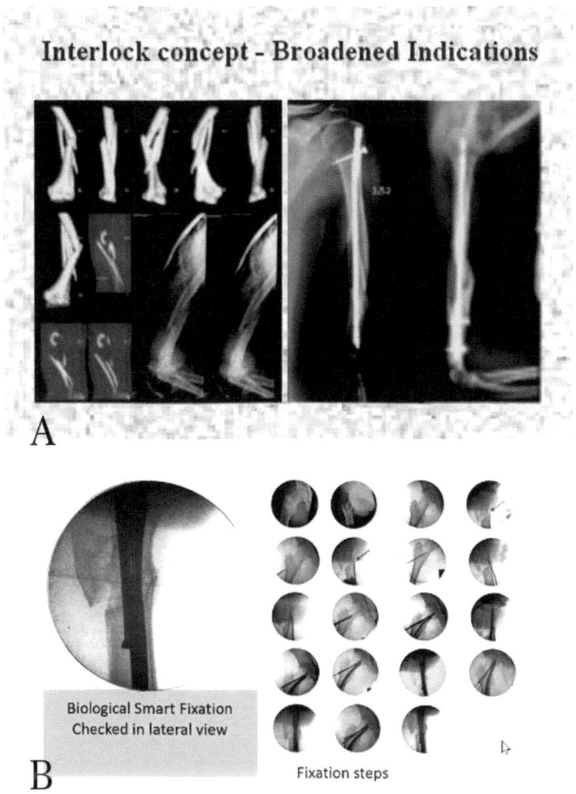

Fig. 10.7 Elaborate compositions. (**a**) X-rays of variety of fracture patterns are arranged in aesthetically pleasing way to explain indications for a technique. (**b**) Image intensifier generated views are collated and processed to create a stunning montage. Such an array is an asset for printed communication where it can be explained in detail and be studied at a suitable pace. Looking at so many images at a go in a live lecture is baffling even for an informed audience. 'Mystification is simple; clarity is the hardest thing of all...'—Julian Barnes

computer generated arrows. One needs to predetermine their need, place, and timing. Arrows can be made to appear and disappear at the required spot and time at a mouse click; this is the only animation recommended in an 8–10 minutes scientific presentation. Block arrows are more visible and are preferred over line arrows.

Only oral consent is necessary to show a patient's X-rays, etc.; however, the identity text must be carefully covered up in each and every instance. Figure 10.9 summarizes refinements of using an X-ray image in medical presentations.

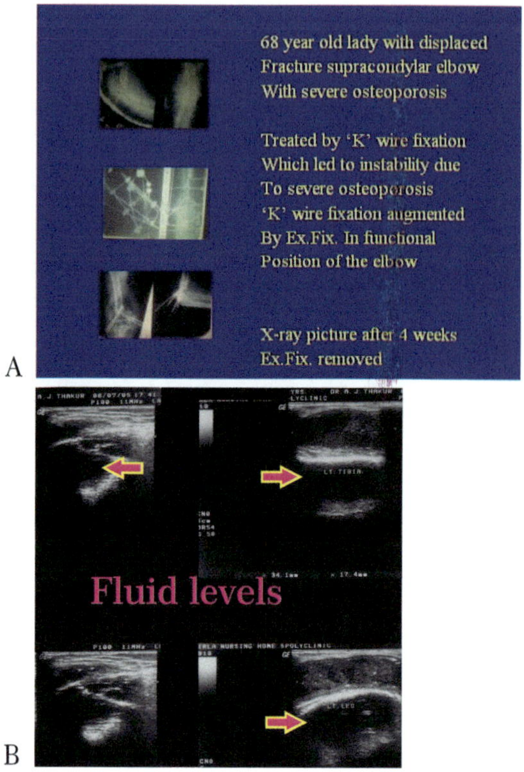

Fig. 10.8 Avoid poor-quality X-rays in a presentation. (**a**) The size and clarity of the X-rays do not add to understanding the problem. (**b**) Sonography film showing fluid level in a bony cavity. Adding text and computer generated block arrows improves lucidity

Fig. 10.9 Summary of all the niceties of showing X-rays, CT, MRI, and USG scans in a medical presentation

X-rays in presentation

Image acquisition

- Use tripod to steady the camera
- Control ambient light
- Focus sharp
- Procure images from workstation and CD

Image modification

- Use only grayscale images
- Crop the redundant area
- Improve brightness and sharpness
- Ethical content modification

Image display

- Avoid insert box
- Amplify image size
- Abhor photomontages
- Avoid poor quality images
- Automated arrows efficient
- Assure patient privacy

Use of Illustrations in Medical Presentations

11

'You are judged on the work you present, not the work you do; always take time to deliver high quality slides'– Anonymous

Contents

Line Drawings

Line drawings have been used to explain a concept or illustrate an object from beginning of the civilization. Photographs, since the advent in the late nineteenth century have tried to replace line drawings. However, graphics and photographs are complementary and not competing media; on several occasions one needs both the elements to make a complete picture. It is rational that both have found their way in medical presentations.

Before use of a computer became commonplace, line drawings were a preserve of a few select people who had the gift of the art of fine drawing. Computer changed the situation and put the fine art of drawing and sketching into the hands of those who are prepared to learn a computer app and produce aesthetically pleasing illustrations.

In learning process people use reading, seeing, and hearing faculties. Between just a picture and picture and text, the later combination is superior for learning; however, people are unenthusiastic to read a lot of on-screen text; a picture and text is superior to animation and on-screen text. People learn and remember best when a

Supplementary Information The online version contains supplementary material available at [https://doi.org/10.1007/978-981-19-1816-2_11].

A. J. Thakur, *Tapping the Power of PowerPoint for Medical Posters and Presentations*, https://doi.org/10.1007/978-981-19-1816-2_11

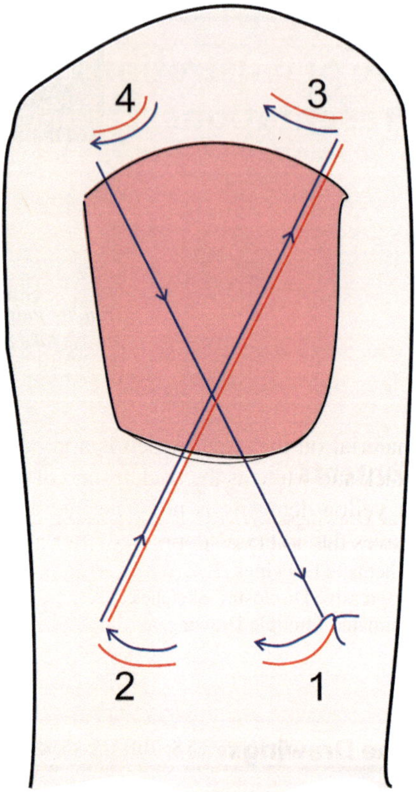

Fig. 11.1 Tension band suture for a fracture of the terminal phalanx. The entire procedure is clearly demonstrated in a simple drawing

talk is accompanied with graphics and as little text on screen as possible; animations have low priority in learning and should be used only if deemed absolutely essential.

Line drawings are used in medical presentations for numerous reasons. A simple sketch can explain the entire procedure at a glance (Fig. 11.1).

Action of a muscle and its effect on a bone segment can be explained in words but a drawing makes it easy to understand (Fig. 11.2). The figure was created in a graphic design app for a presentation.

Explaining a technique in steps, a figure helps to clarify the finer points (Fig. 11.3).

Photographs and Drawings

Photographs are excellent medium to show the details of an object. When the function of the object is to be explained, addition of a figure goes a long way (Fig. 11.4).

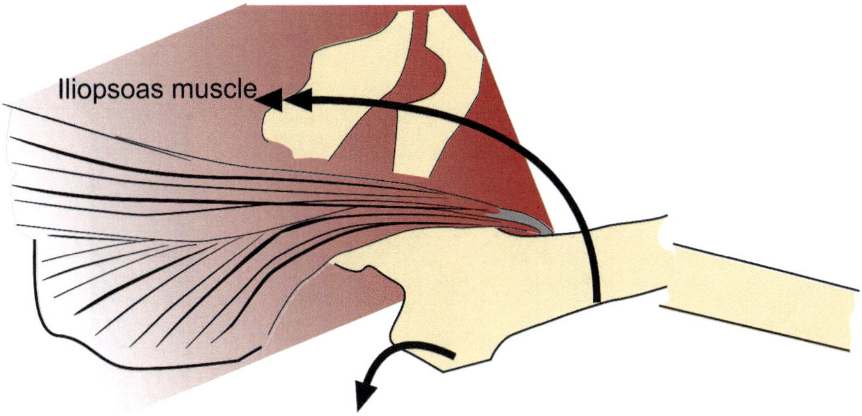

Fig. 11.2 Muscle action. Action of Iliopsoas muscle displaces the fractured proximal femur is shown graphically

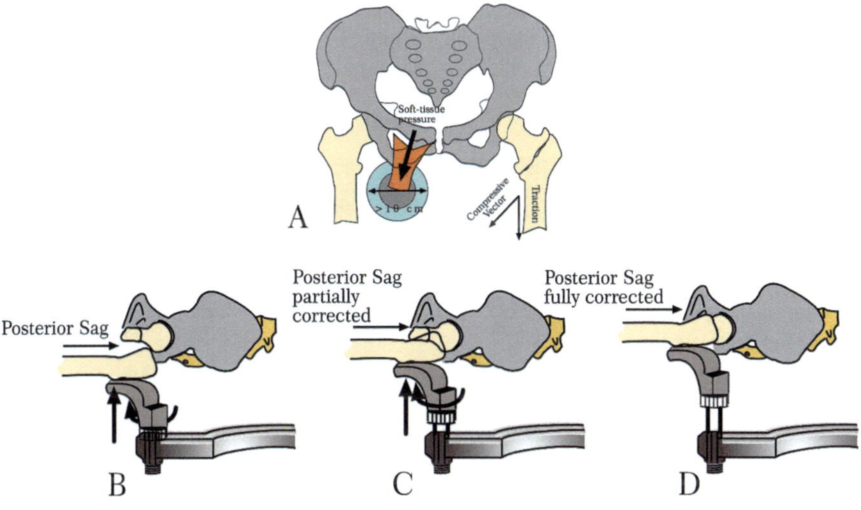

Fig. 11.3 Step by step exposé. (**a**) The main features of the traction are illustrated in this section (**b**) A finer point of reduction is highlighted. (**c** and **d**) show the active solution

Value of a photograph is enhanced by adding a few sketches. Figure 11.5 shows a positioning photograph for mortice view of an ankle. Adding a sketch of X-ray tube, its rays and drawing a couple of reference lines on the photograph makes it more meaningful. It now prompts to rotate the foot or incline the X-ray tube to get the desired view.

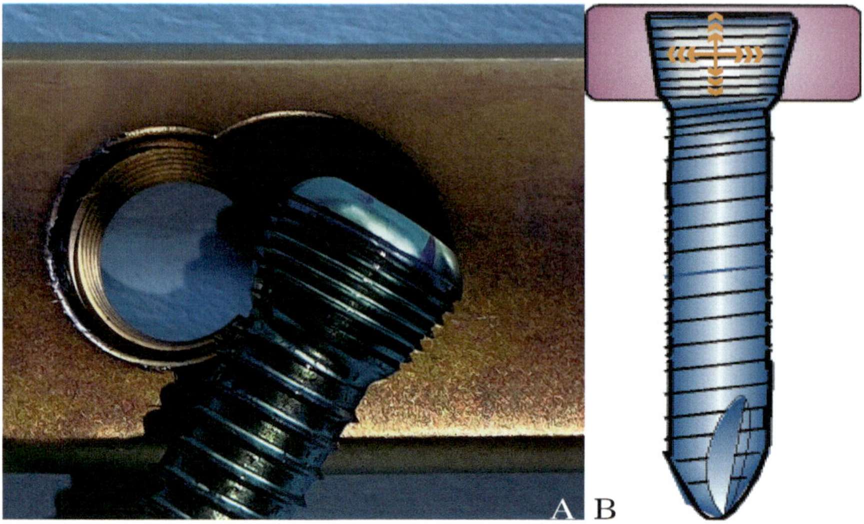

Fig. 11.4 Photograph of a locking plate. (**a**) A well focused photograph shows all the details of a plate's design but does not give any idea of its working. (**b**) A sketch showing the screw-plate in cross section with arrows conveys an interaction between the threads in the plate and those on the screw head and alludes to their functionality

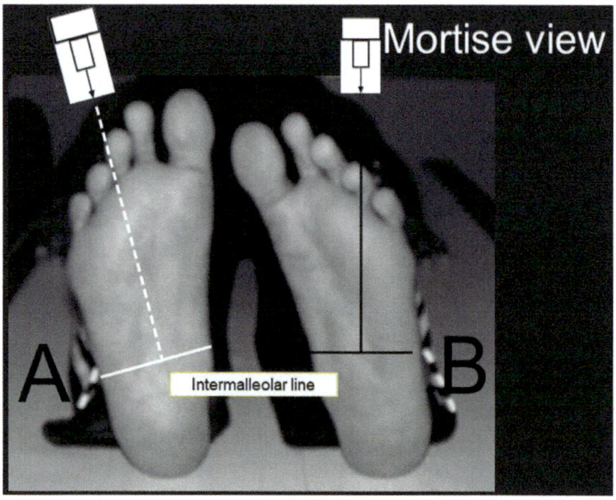

Fig. 11.5 Positioning photograph for mortice view of the ankle. Without addition of the figure of X-ray tube, marking the probable angle of the X-rays and anatomical reference lines, the photograph offers little information

Schematic Drawings

A body cell has several components; some of them cannot be visualized even by electron microscope at a given time. However, all the information about a body cell can be illustrated in a drawing (Fig. 11.6).

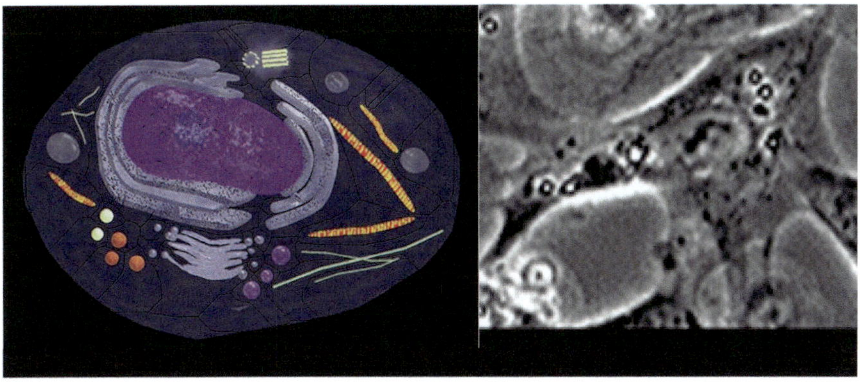

A B

Fig. 11.6 Two images of a body cell. (**a**) A simplified diagram showing internal structures of a body cell. (**b**) Electron microscopic photograph does not show all the structures of a cell in one view

Progressive Disclosure Sketches

Journey of an ovum from ovary down the fallopian tube can be progressively shown in a set of 16 slides or schematically summarized in a single one (Fig. 11.7). Sketches and progressive disclosure helps in understanding a process (Video 11.1).

Several features of a small object can only be emphasized by using a fully labelled diagram (Fig. 11.8).

It is difficult to understand how a drill cuts the material. Use of a line diagram clearly visualizes the mechanism (Fig. 11.9).

Animated Multiple Drawings

Multiple drawings are made in a graphic design program and used to compose a scene in a presentation program (Fig. 11.10). All the individual drawings are moved to create an informative animated sequence resembling a video.

Presentation programs have limited drawing capabilities. All the illustrations displayed here are made in a stand-alone graphic app to get the desired effect. Use of drawings in a presentation should be selective; drawings may be used only when needed to make a point and the figure must relate to the message. Each displayed figure must make the message clearer otherwise it becomes a source of distraction. There should be no unnecessary figure in a presentation, like a machine should not have an unnecessary nut or bolt. Each drawing should be modified to retain only the relevant part and other unnecessary segment should be covered or removed; the applicable element of the illustration may be redrawn for clarity and elegance; help of an artist is recommended in this context. Graphics that come with the presentation app are overused. It is better to search for new figures on the web where large

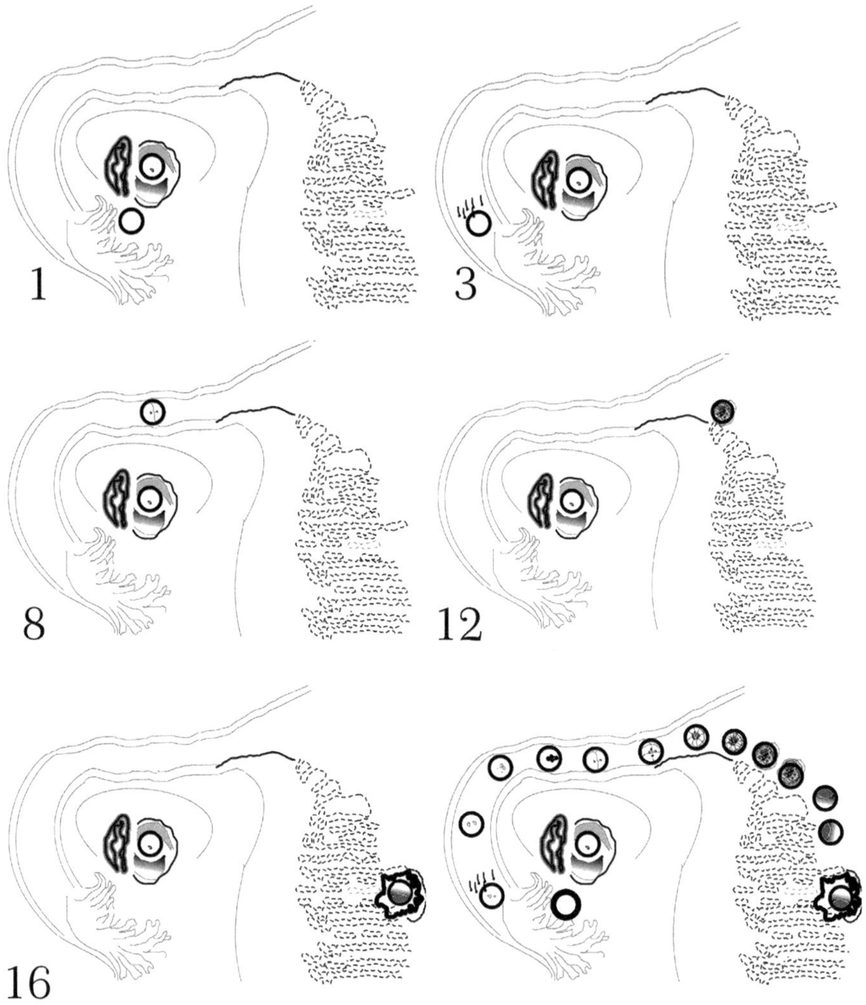

Fig. 11.7 Passage of a fertilized ovum through the fallopian tube. The slides are serially numbered; a few are shown here. Inset. A single slide can show the entire passage

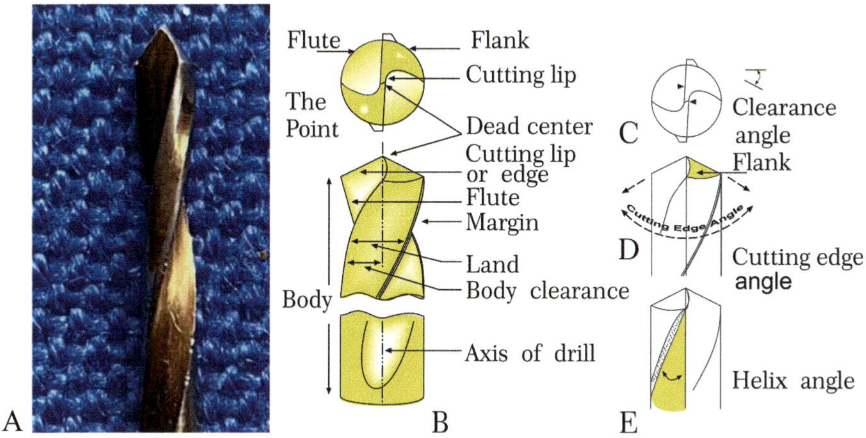

Fig. 11.8 Drill bit. (**a**) Photograph shows salient features of a drill bit. (**b**–**e**) show all the relevant details of the tool underlining the importance of a drawing in a medical presentation

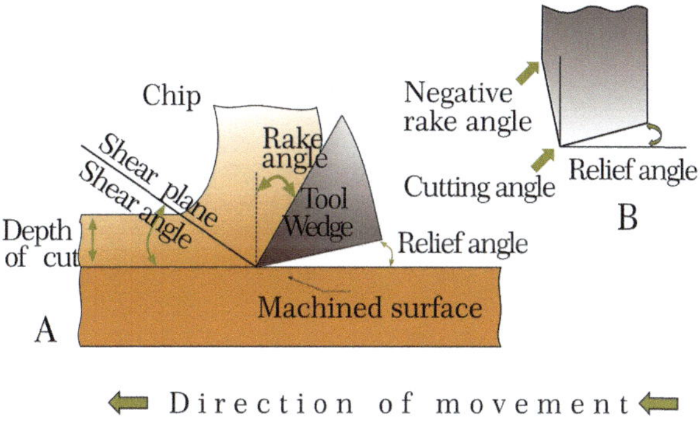

Fig. 11.9 Cutting action of a sharp tool. (**a**) Illustration explains the action of the cutting edge of a tool (**b**) Finer points of the mechanism are elucidated

Fig. 11.10 Drawings for animation. Several separate figures are created in a drawing program and assembled on a slide of a presentation program. Using its animation feature these are moved in a meaningful way to convey a message

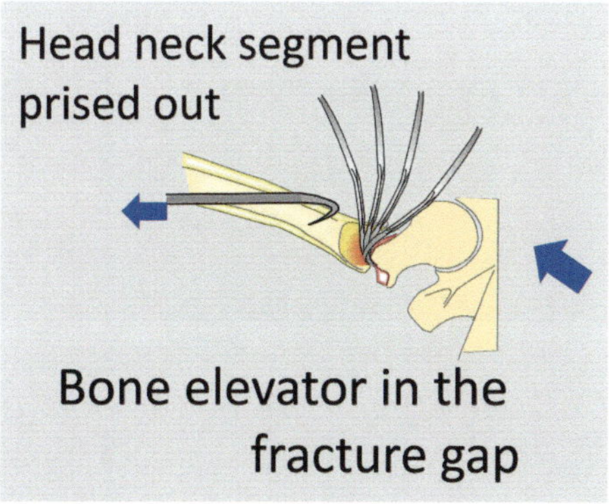

number of illustrations, line drawings, clipart are available; pictures can also be borrowed from printed literature. Whatever the source of a diagram, copyright must be respected.

Graphics are powerful tools to get a message across. Computers make it easy to access illustrations in large numbers. Relevant and quality figures make an impact while worthless sketches damage the objective of a presentation.

Adding Videos in Presentations 12

A picture tells a thousand words, and video footage tells millions.– Tang, Shou-jiang, Raju, Gottumukkala

Contents

Digital photography includes videography. Digital and phone cameras are capable of recording videos. Guidelines for patient's consent for recoding video are similar to ones for photography. Taking a video is also similar to taking a photograph and some of the technical necessities have been discussed in Chap. 9.

Video Formats

Video's resolutions are steadily increasing, the file size also grows and could be large and awkward to use. Programs called Codecs compress the raw video data by encoding and compacting it for storing and sharing. Codecs are used again to decode that data to decompress it for editing and viewing. H.264 or AVC are popular codecs for this purpose. Videos have several constituents that must be put together in to the final parcel (Fig. 12.1). The components needed for reviewing the video are actual video portion, additional files like audio, text sub-titles, synchronization

A. J. Thakur, *Tapping the Power of PowerPoint for Medical Posters and Presentations*, https://doi.org/10.1007/978-981-19-1816-2_12

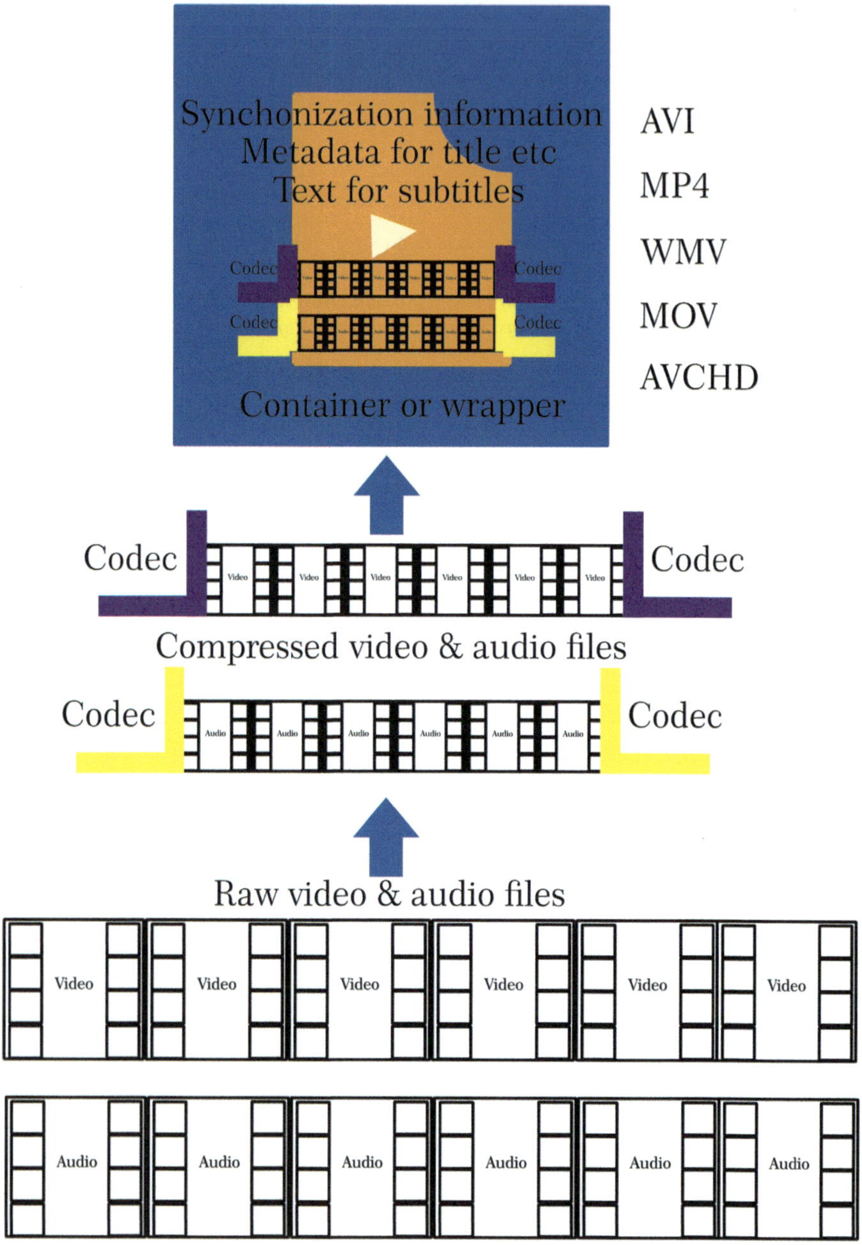

Fig. 12.1 File format explained. Construction of a common file format for viewing a video is shown

information, and metadata such as title; all these elements must be together. Audio file formats or file extensions are the containers or wrappers to keep together these elements of the video. The common formats are:

MP4

MP4 (MPEG-4 Part 14) is a popular video file format. It can play on most devices. This format works well for videos posted on YouTube, Facebook, Twitter, and Instagram.

MOV

MOV (QuickTime Film) files tend to be quite large. It uses MPEG-4 encoding to play in QuickTime Player for Windows. MOV is supported by Facebook and YouTube and it works well for TV viewing.

WMV

WMV (Windows Media Viewer) files are also large in size like MOV. YouTube supports WMV and Apple owners can view these videos by using Windows Media Player for Apple.

AVI

AVI (Audio Video Interleave) works in almost all situations. AVI offers the highest quality but also large file sizes. It is supported by YouTube and works well for TV viewing.

AVCHD

Advanced Video Coding High Definition is built for Panasonic and Sony digital camcorders; these files compress for easy storage without losing definition.

Playing a video file will sometimes require the user to install a codec file corresponding to the type of video and audio coding used in the file. FFmpeg is a free software that has a large collection of Codecs and of programs for editing video, audio, and other multimedia files. VLC Media Player can run almost any video file.

Acquisition of a Video

Acquisition of a video for medical presentation with a quality cell phone camera or a digital camera is an acceptable approach. Whenever possible the camera should be mounted on a stand during shooting to avoid minor hand movements. The subject should be in adequate light. The videos for medical presentation should always be recorded in a landscape view; rotating a video shot in portrait view does not show well in presentation app.

Clinical videos may be recorded at a permanent site in the hospital; a neutral background works well. In operation theatre the main lights are too bright for video recording and should be dimmed or switched off. Video should be recorded using prevailing ambient light. Record–pause–record sequence is recommended when covering a surgical procedure; Video unfolds a story and it is essential to preplan the sequence. Continuous recording is wasteful because one is unable to use a large segment for presentation. It is a good practice to shoot simultaneously a few still photographs of the subject; they come handy on a rainy day. A frame copied from a video is not as sharp as an original photograph.

Inserting a Video in a Presentation

The recorded videos should be modified in an editing program to suit the purpose of medical presentation. Short videos are effective in making a point. The running length of the video could be adjusted in the presentation program itself but at times use of a stand-alone video editing app is required. In presentation, one should use videos judiciously. Like too many photographs or X-rays, too many videos in a presentation are counterproductive. One need not show everything that one has in one go. Inserting a video in a presentation app needs special attention. Each presentation program has a method to import a video; it should be meticulously followed. All the presentation programs offer an option of running the video automatically or on click. 'Automatic' is the best choice. Whenever a video is run 'on a click', there is lag between the click and video running; the anticipative lull is agonizing for the speaker as well as the audience. Automatic running of multiple videos on a slide can also be fine-tuned by arranging animation sequences. Such an arrangement is beneficial because always there is lag after each click to start the video which breaks the speaker's link and is unsettling for the audience. A running video can be 'paused and run' by using keyboard shortcuts or mouse clicks.

Video Playback Fiasco

The presentation app does not embed large videos; at the appropriate time it links up with the video file. The size of the presentation file remains small with this mechanism; very large files slow down the projection process. A computer can easily link up if the video file is in the same folder. An inserted video will not run in a presentation if the video file is not available on the conference computer. Although presentation programs offer 'embed video' option, it is safer to copy the video in the folder and carry it with you than to blame a technical failure. It is unsound practice to stretch a video to make it larger on the screen. This adversely affects its quality and slows down the playback. If there are several videos in a presentation, then one should contact the organizers well in time with a request to either make special arrangements for a powerful computer with relevant software or grant permission to present from a personal computer.

The other important cause of failure to show a video is codec mismatch. Every camera maker has its own codec which is not compatible with other systems. This causes difficulties in running the videos on computers that do not carry the required codec. It helps to convert the video for presentation to formats that are almost universal, e.g. AVI, MP4, WMV, and MOV. Video format converters are freely available on the web and should be used.

Transporting a Video

Carrying a presentation with a video sequence to a conference always needs extra precautions. It is a safe practice to copy every inserted video file to a folder along with the presentation file. This folder should be copied to two portable storage devices and carried to the conference; as an insurance, the folder should also be available on the cloud.

Complexities of video software are outside the comfort zone of healthcare professionals; it is a good practice to test every video in the preview room. The audiovisual team of the meeting may be able to sort out the issues if there is time on hand; it is embarrassing to announce on the stage that the video is not working due to technicalities.

Avoid Videos

Web offers several video-sharing sites where videos of every description are available for download. This situation tempts people to download and show low-quality clips in the presentations. Many feel such inclusion may turn their presentation more interesting, lively, or create light moments in otherwise serious milieu. More often these clips are irrelevant to the topic, only offer entertainment and have no educational value. A wise presenter should steer clear of the temptation to use such videos.

13 Posters for Medical & Scientific Meetings

'Delegates whose abstracts for oral presentations are not selected will be invited to display and discuss their research in a poster presentation'. – stereotypical notification in a conference brochure

Contents

History of Poster Presentation

The poster presentation had a 'rejected' feeling about it. And this was not without reason. One of the largest organizers of scientific information, the American Heart Association (AHA) in 1974, first began considering poster sessions as an effective and inexpensive technique for presenting research when requests for simultaneous

A. J. Thakur, *Tapping the Power of PowerPoint for Medical Posters and Presentations*, https://doi.org/10.1007/978-981-19-1816-2_13

traditional sessions exceeded conference space and time constraints. In 1976, the AHA approved poster session as a one-off trial when 180 abstracts were accepted as posters, on the basis of their scientific merit. In 2000, nearly 50% of abstracts, or about 3000 posters were approved and presented at AHA's annual scientific conference. Other associations and learned societies picked up the trend and conducted poster sessions ranging from 10 to over 13,000 presentations at a single conference. In India, the poster sessions began because of similar reasons—time and space constraints—in the Silver Jubilee Conference of Indian Orthopaedic Association held in 1980 at Mumbai. No longer a destination for 'oral rejects', organizers of prestigious meetings now 'invite' abstracts for posters and select a few for display; poster abstracts are now a part of conference proceedings and are counted as publications. Scientific meetings in medicine, nursing, and allied health specialities widely use poster presentations and now it is one of the regular formats to present research at a such conferences.

What Is a Poster Presentation?

Poster is a useful tool to introduce new unpublished scientific data. It is an opportunity for young investigators to test their work in real time, receive quick feedback in a nonthreatening and collegial environment as their presence is required near the poster. It is an opportunity to be more speculative and to say more than one could say in conventional literature. Feedback received during a poster session helps in refining the research and in preparing it for publication in a peer reviewed journal. Poster session interactions can forge new contacts and create new job opportunities. Preparing and defending a poster hones an investigator's presentation skills. Usually only titles or at most the abstracts of the posters are considered published in conference proceedings which receive wide distribution.

A poster is a visual presentation of a research or clinical project. Its appeal is through visuals and graphics as it uses schematic diagrams, graphs, tables, and other strategies to direct viewer's visual attention; text is less important. A poster is not a mini-journal article; several posters appear as cut and paste version of a manuscript and put off visitors who are reluctant to read and find out what is it about. A poster may be treated as an advertisement of a research project; visual appeal plays a dominant role in attracting a scientific visitor. A poster may report a descriptive, observational, retrospective, or experimental study; or evaluate a method, a device, or a protocol; or present a case series or a single case report. The purpose of creating a poster will dictate its content; is it intended to engage the attendees in a discussion or collaborate in the ongoing research? Is it just to present knowledge for others to benefit?—answers to such questions will decide the content of a poster.

Poster displays salient features of a study; it often is a prelude to a scientific article. It is a semiofficial declaration of results before it is submitted for a peer review by a journal. Poster carries only highlights of a study; details of the study appear in a scientific article. A scientific article on the other side is a self-supporting entity; it is read leisurely without time restriction. This difference in reading time availability allows the article to carry more detailed text and graphics; the tables and graphs in an article could be considered in depth and at leisure. A poster has a short life. Posters are set up in a prominent place in the conference complex. A specified time, 45–60 minutes, is marked when the presenter is expected to standby his creation and conference attendees come by to see and may discuss some issues. 'The cardinal sin of poster presenters … is...they assume people are going to stand there and read the posters in silence for 10 straight minutes, following the order of the sections they have laid out', (Anonymous). It is estimated that an attendee views a poster for 10 seconds from a distance of 10 feet (3 metres). It means the decision to stop or move on is made in 4–6 seconds. A poster is also viewed when the author is not present. A poster must be eye-catching and striking as there are several other posters competing for attention. A good balance between large graphics and text attracts visitors.

Abstract

Conference organizers invite abstracts for poster presentations; often when they cannot accommodate a submission for oral presentation offer an opportunity to present the research in poster format. Preparing an abstract is an art by itself. A prospective presenter must adapt to the specifications provided by the meeting organizers to avoid automatic disqualification. Abstract describing new and original data stands better chance of acceptance compared to a previously published or presented work; a well-written scholarly piece, complete studies, studies with some promise, good statistical workout, sound methodology stand good chance of acceptance. Acceptance of an abstract for poster presentation means very little. Conferences needs attendees and revenue. Time for oral presentation is at a premium. Poster acceptance opens up an official avenue to attend a conference for many attendees. However, one needs to work on the poster to get academic advantage of the opportunity.

Abstract is a precis of the research work and has many uses. The conference organizers use it to select a poster for presentation. It is browsed by many attendees before deciding to visit a poster. The abstracts are placed on the conference website and is picked by search engines; these are also printed in conference handouts and published as conference proceedings. The organizers may specify a word limit whether formatted or unformatted. An abstract should state in a lucid language the significance and purpose of the study, explain what was done and what was found and finally sum-up what it means. It should include searchable keywords and be devoid of abbreviations, ambiguous references, or phrases.

Pre-Poster Planning

Horses for courses; a poster should be suitable for the anticipated audience. Who will visit the poster?—established clinicians or medical students; residents or nurses. New researchers, and seasoned scientists will have different needs and poster should cater to that. In most large meetings the attendees would be a mix of different categories. Such information will dictate the level of background material, text, and graphics. One should include what is most relevant to the audience.

Size Requirements

It is important to know the required size of the poster for a conference. The size may vary from organization to organization. The American Academy of Orthopaedic Surgeons prefers posters of 114.3 cm × 114.3 cm dimension. Other common size is 106.6 cm × 142.2 cm; alternatively, 91.4 × 142.2 cm would provide an aspect ratio of 16:9. Bombay Orthopaedic Society's WIROC® (Western India Regional Orthopaedic Conference) needs posters to be of 122 cm × 61 cm which is a common size in India. It is tedious to resize a poster once the centrepieces are in place. A poster of an incorrect dimension is likely to be rejected or may stand out for wrong reasons.

Classification of Posters

A poster's outline can be of two types.

1. Type 1

   A poster is prepared on conventional lines—IMRaD—Introduction, Method, Results, and Discussion (Fig. 13.1). The title is included in the banner along with the names of the author, institution, and other standard information. Background or rationale statement introduces the theme of the poster and is followed by the research questions or hypothesis. How the study was carried out is put down under material and methods. Only the broad moves should be mentioned in a bulleted format. This includes the approach taken to answer the scientific question with mention of the sample—population's background, selection criteria, and group assignment—interventions used and statistical methods used. Too many details of the method may slow down the visitor so it should be provided in a handout. Observation of the experiments follow under results heading which attracts wide attention. Use of graphics to report results is superior to a narrative. Tables may be used sparingly, with minimum of embedded text. Simple figures with explanatory labelling are very effective. Conclusions are important and are mentioned in bulleted format for easy reading and grasp. Important acknowledgements, funding details, conflict of interest statement, and contact details bring up the rear.

   Scientific posters are meant to be skimmed, not read in detail. Abstract and discussion are often omitted in a poster. Abstract is circulated to the attendees before the conference and does not add anything but occupies valuable space and slows down the reader. Discussion in brief is not useful, and is often omitted in a poster and given out in a handout. Although a manuscript's format—IMRaD—is followed the text is greatly reduced and most often bulleted text is presented. Figures, graphics, and charts are used to illustrate and reduce the need for text. A right mix of text, figures, and colour is aimed to make the poster attractive.

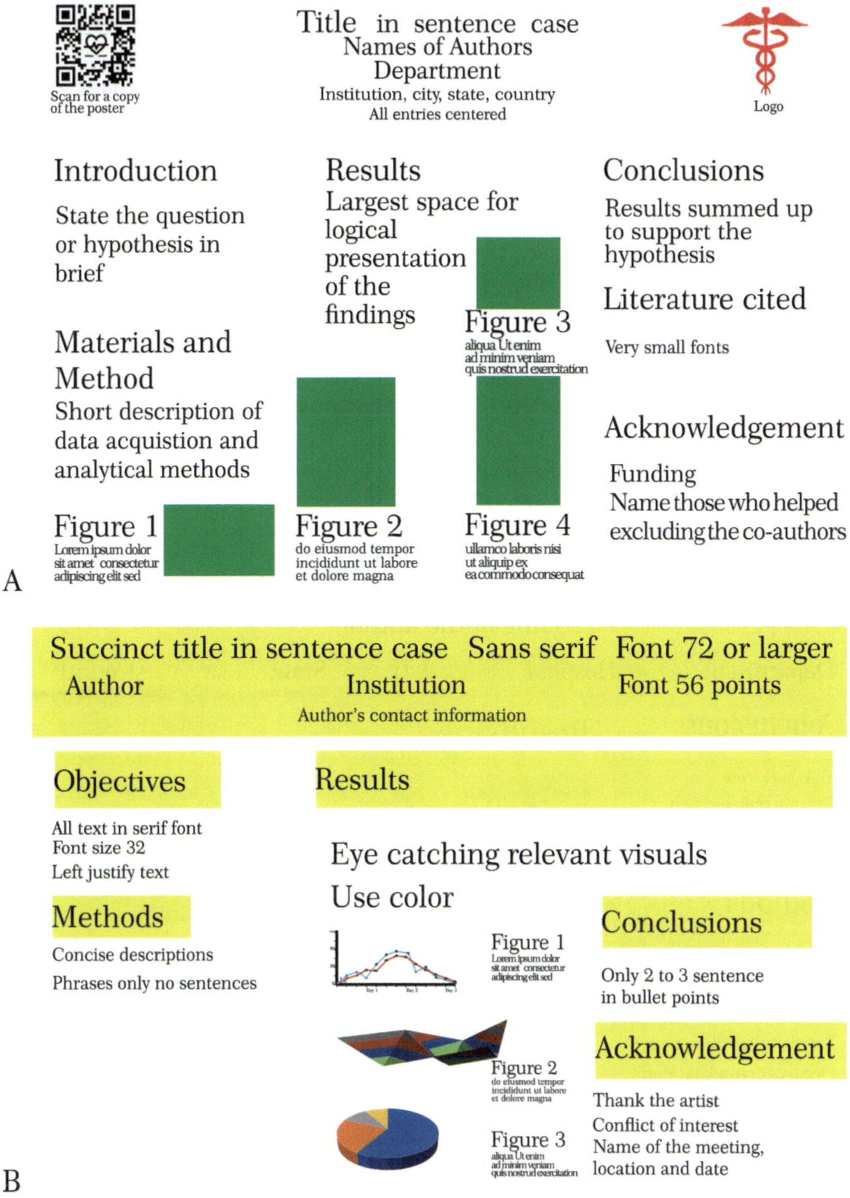

Fig. 13.1 Posters following established format of presenting scientific material. There is neither enough place on the poster for discussion nor the conference attendee has enough time to read it. Everyone is interested in conclusions and these should be prominently displayed. (**a**) QR code facilitates easy dispersal of large quantity of related information. (**b**) Use of appropriate font size ensures a poster's legibility while use of high-quality graphics captures a visitor's attention

2. Type II

After reading the title, a visitor to the poster area looks at the upper left corner; the most important information ought to be here. What did the study find out? How is it affecting the reader? This information is always found in the conclusion section at the bottom right corner. The matters that are normally conveyed in the bottom line should be presented in the most visited spot, the upper left corner (Fig. 13.2). Conclusions should be presented in a bulleted format. The next important thing in a poster is the results section. Results are best expressed in graphs, figures, and photos; explanatory text should be either embedded in or be near the figure or data. Humans learn more when clarifying text is combined with visual information. Minimum text should be used to present results. There is no place for decorative images in a poster as they distract a reader. Methods come next and be expressed as flow charts or graphics with minimum instructive text included in them. The details of the methods are not expected here; it may be given in a handout or conveyed orally to an enquiring visitor. Presenter needs to be bold and not follow the beaten old style of poster. Poster is like an advertisement board for the research. If it is off beat in a nice and useful way then no

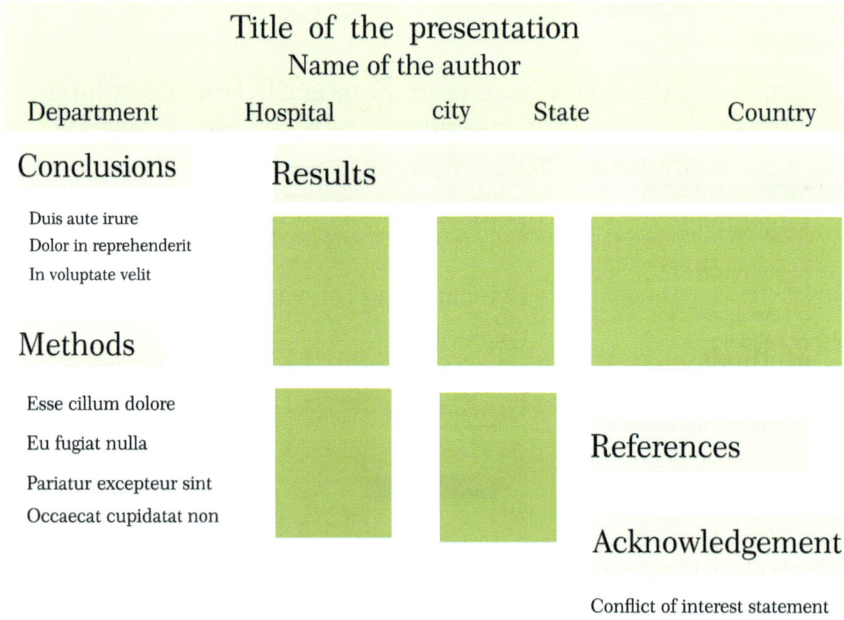

Fig. 13.2 Evidence from advertising and psychology suggests that a visitor to a poster makes up his mind in 10 seconds to stay or move on. He uses up to 6 seconds to read the title and then scans the upper left corner of the poster for next 4 seconds to know what happened to the stated question or hypothesis; he seeks the answer in conclusions. When the conclusions are presented in upper left corner in short bulleted sentences the information is understood promptly by the attendee. If the evidence is useful, then the visitor will look for figures, graphs, or photos which are widely spread out under results. When all this is of use, then the visitor pays attention to method and other headings before engaging with the presenter

one, including the judges would mind the change; it may even set a trend. Increasing number of organizers are asking for funding details and conflict of interest statements. Discussion and references may be added in the space at the bottom end of the poster or better still, they be included in the handouts.

Layout of a Poster

A poster may be in landscape or portrait format. It should be visually attractive. White space—area without any printing is important factor in making a poster attractive. Around 35% of the poster should be left as white space. The material on the poster should be arranged by following 'axis of symmetry'; the text and graphics are placed symmetrically across a central horizontal, vertical, or diagonal axis. A poster should have a margin of 3 cm all around.

A Poster's Title

The title is included in poster's banner. A poster addresses one central question which when clearly stated, provides a clear and explicit take-home message. The question should be posed in the title. Title is the only thing the visitors can read from a distance and should be like a visual bait, to attract people to come close to look at other details in the poster. The title should be eye-catching like a newspaper headline. It may pose a question, announce the scope of the study, or allude to a new finding. Short, sharp, and compelling are a few attributes of a good title. Two-part title separated by a colon is in vogue. This device is used to add more information and at times, gentle humour. 'your poster needs to be beautiful, with a very short and attractive, meaningful title'. – Anonymous.

The names of authors, institutional affiliations come next. Institutional logo is a big thing for many presenters and should be placed here. Banner is also the place for QR code, if so desired. Use of QR code facilitates quick access to vast quantities of information. A QR code is the 'next step' for those who are interested in knowing more about the poster's contents. In place of writing down the contact telephone or email address, copying a QR code takes the visitor to the presenter's website, or social media account and provides more information and a permanent contact point. QR code could be a link to presenter's supplementary data, ORCID iD, LinkedIn, or ResearchGate profiles. Institutional logo can be added to the centre of the QR code. The QR code needs to be big enough to be able to scan from a metre away. It is a good practice to state the destination, e.g. 'scan here to download the paper' linking to a full version of the study and a copy of the poster. QR code is 'stupidly easy' to make and serves conference attendees who take pictures of posters, better.

The 'sweet spot' in the poster is the top left corner. After looking at the banner at the top of the poster with the title and other essentials, a visitor then tracks to the upper left corner. Most important information should be placed here. A summary or abstract is often placed here. But most readers are in a hurry, after reading the title, are keen to know the conclusions drawn from the study. It is a bit odd to place the end piece of the study at the beginning but is the most satisfying read for the attendee. If conclusions are placed here in readable bulleted text and are appealing, then a visitor is likely to take more interest in the poster and the presenter.

What comes next depends on which pattern of presentation is being used, i.e. type I or II. Results are best expressed in graphics with embedded text for 'clear portrayal of complexity'. Chunks of text arranged in paragraphs are most likely to be overlooked; text in bulleted pattern has best chance of being read. Results should have the highest number of graphs and tables. Simple tables with minimal explanatory icons are preferred over a detailed, text heavy tables from a paper published in print. General outline of method followed is enough in a poster. Greater detail can be provided in a handout or via QR code. Infographics may be used to introduce both results and method in a poster. Infographics are visual representation of information, data, or knowledge for quick and clear dispersal. These are designed with minimum assumptions about the readers' knowledge base. Infographics improve understanding by using figures to see patterns and trends.

Medical fraternity is in an era of open disclosure. It is expected of every researcher to disclose fully their connections with industry or any other entity who has funded the research or is likely to influence judgement due to conflict of interest. This has become an essential component for posters presented at several leading medical conferences. This information should be voluntarily and truthfully disclosed because it helps the attendees to judge and determine the impact of bias on the presented research.

Steps of Poster Construction

A brief account of nuances of poster construction follows.

Background

Text placed on a light background is easy to read. A light background with dark letters is the natural way we read a newspaper; images and graphs also stand out against light background. This arrangement is specially applicable for dermatology posters who have a greater share of images. Certain themes in posters can dictate colour choice—for example, a pink colour may suit posters dealing with paediatric subjects. Some dyslexic individuals relate better to a poster printed on a cream, or off-white, good quality matt paper.

Lettering

The lettering in the title should be large. 100-point lettering can be read from 4.5 metres. General recommendations for font sizes in a poster are: the names of the author and associates in 56 points; other materials like department, name of the institution, etc., in 40 points. All headings in 48 points while sub-headings in 36 points to attract the reader. The entire text in 32–36 points. The letters in these font sizes are easy to read from a distance (Fig. 13.3).

Fancy typefaces must not be used. The typeface for a poster should be chosen with care. A combination of two typefaces, one for title/headings and one for the body text makes an appealing display (Fig. 13.4). Underlining the text for emphasis

	Point	Legibility distance
Title	72 to 150	72 point font is legible at 4. 2 meters
Authors	56	56 point font is legible at 3.6 meters
Heading	48	48 point font is legible at 3 meters Should be easily readable for anyone walking nearby
Subheading	36	36 point font is legible at 2.1 meters
Main body text	32	32 point font is legible at 1.5 meters
Captions	24	24 point font is legible at 1.3 meters

Fig. 13.3 A quick guide to the size of the letters to ensure satisfactory legibility of the poster from a distance

Typeface combinations

Title	Body
Corbel	Clarendon Lt BT
Bodoni	Futura
Clarendon BT	Futura
Franklin Gothic	Baskerville
Arial	Times New Roman
Gadugi	Century 751 BT

Don't use fancy fonts

Fig. 13.4 A combination of serif and sans serif typefaces appears attractive on a poster. Fancy typefaces have no place in medical and scientific posters creates cluttered appearance; the line obscures the descender strokes of the letters and diminishes their identification values; instead, bold or italic fonts may be used. Text should be in sentence case; text in all capitals is hard to read. Similarly light letters on dark background are also difficult to read. Dark letters on light background are easiest to follow. Text printed in yellow does not make an impact. The title, section heading, and sub-heading should be in boldface and the rest of the text should be in regular font.

A poster may be in landscape mode but, the text should not run the entire length of the poster, except in the banner area (Fig. 13.5). It is uncomfortable to read long text line from left to right. Large blocks of text are also intimidating to read while on the move or standing; same material in bullet points appear more friendly, easy to read and understand.

One should use columns and headers, like in a newspaper (Fig. 13.6). Language of the poster should be simple and conversational to describe bare essentials, the guiding tenets being 'simplify language, reduce sentence complexity, and eliminate extraneous details'. All the available space may not be filled; offsetting data with blank (white) spaces makes a poster attractive. A balance is needed as too little white space creates a jumbled look and too much of it makes a poster look empty. Alignment, balance, and spacing are critical in poster's appeal. All contents, headings, columns, graphs, figures, and diagrams should be aligned to bring off aesthetically pleasing appearance. Left-justified text is comfortable to read.

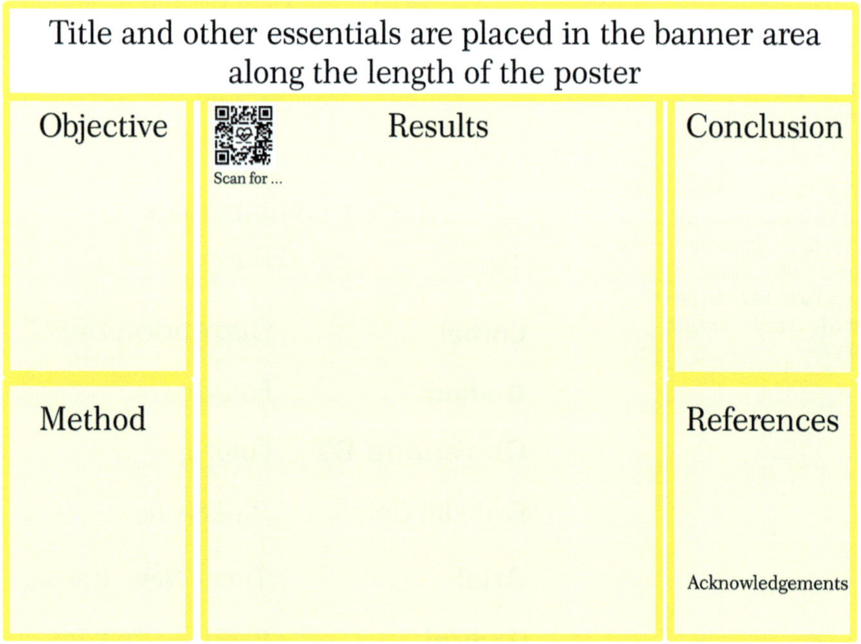

Fig. 13.5 Short text lines with bullets ensure their perusal by attendees who are often rushed to see several posters in a short time

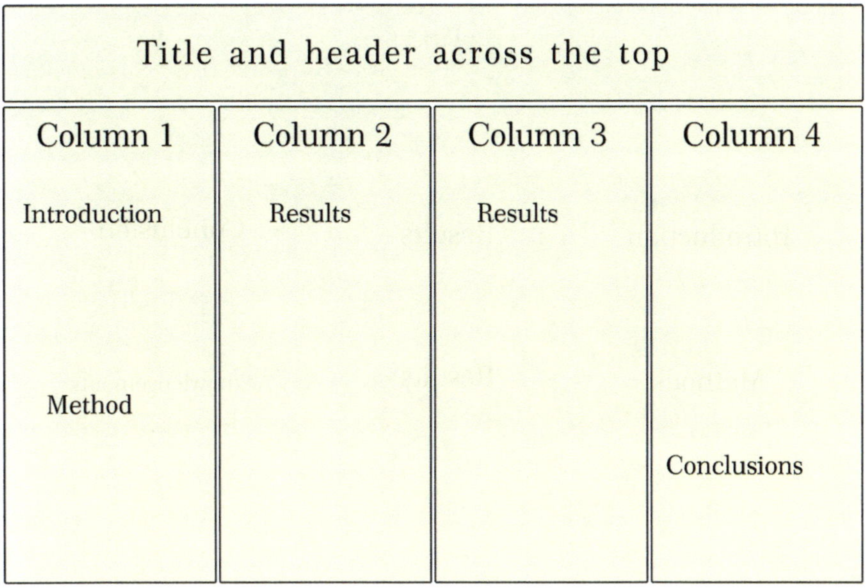

Fig. 13.6 Newspaper style layout is an effective format for a poster

Use of Colour

Colour makes a poster attractive but its use should be restrained (Fig. 13.7). Colour creates a contrast between text and background. Two or three colours are adequate. Overuse of very bright colours initially attracts the viewers but later wear out their eyes, is distracting and annoying; flashy posters do not become a scientific communication.

Cueing Devices

Viewers by force of habit, read from left to right and from top to bottom. They should be guided by using the cueing or signalling devices like numbering, bolding, highlighting, arrows, asterisks, or any other mechanism to move from one logical step to another (Fig. 13.8). Individual creativity may be used to do this guiding in an unusual and eye-catching way.

Graphics

Decorative images should be avoided as they only distract and add nothing to the content. Charts, drawings, radiographs, clinical photographs, paintings and even relevant cartoons increase a poster's appeal. Illustrations make it easy to show

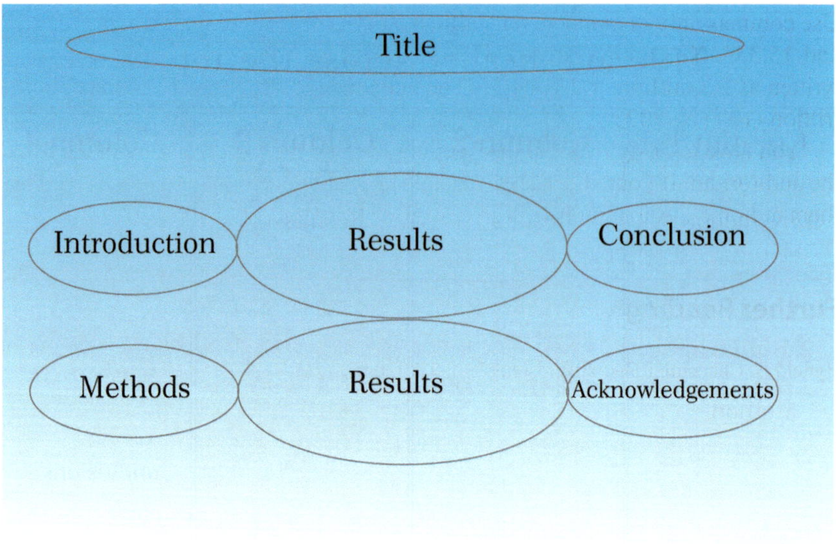

A

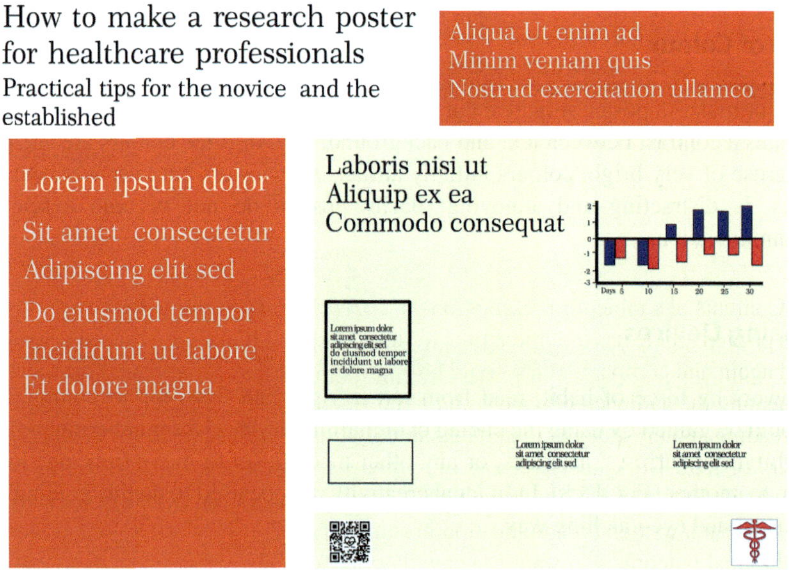

B

Fig. 13.7 Use of colour in poster is welcome but should be restrained. (**a**) Single coloured background offsets the oval shaped text containers (**b**) Colour blocks interspersed with white space appears attractive leaving large space for results

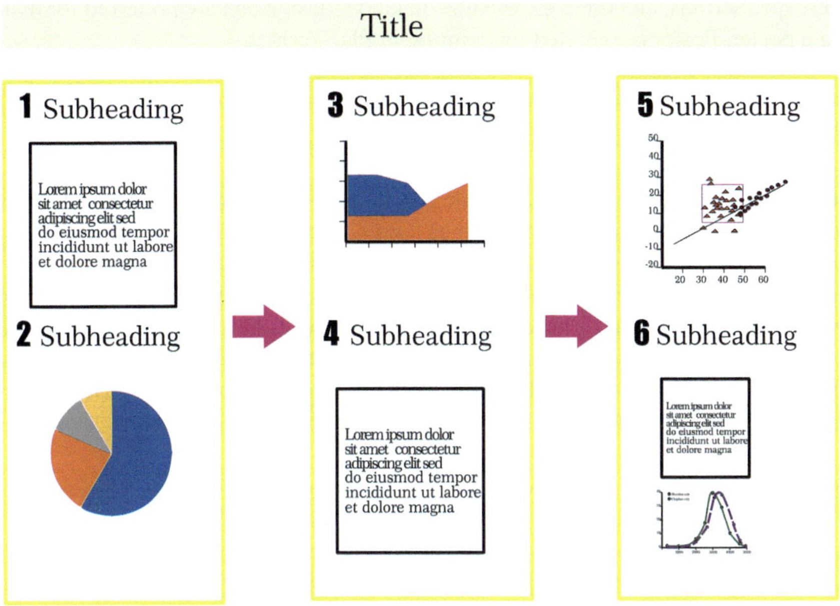

Fig. 13.8 Numbering, bolding, and arrows are some of the devices that guide a reader through a poster

complex concepts, structures, processes, procedures, and methods. The choice of graphics depends on the data at hand. The discussion in Chap. 8 may be referred to make a decision. Illustrations should be clear and well proportioned. Gridlines, 3D graphs, and background colour in a graph result in a cluttered appearance.

Graphs should be simple, consistent in scale, adequately labelled, and big enough to be legible from 1.5 metres. Free downloaded images pixilate and rarely look good on the poster; PNG or TIFF formats are less prone to pixilation. Image resizing by dragging the nodes may distort it; use of resizing tools of a graphic program is recommended. Photographs are not commonly included in research posters, but are more often included in posters setting out case reports. Photographs are used only if they contribute in explaining or emphasizing the message. Photographs should not be copy-pasted but be saved and imported in the poster file. Every diagram, photograph, and graph should be labelled. Refer to every figure in the text for providing context. Photo images are printed at 150–200 dpi and graphics at 225 dpi.

Making a Poster

A poster is made on a computer. PowerPoint has easy to use facility to make one. A poster made on PC may not show well on a Mac and vice versa; there may be display inconsistencies in fonts, colours, and medial file compatibility. Apps like

Inkscape, Scribus, and LaTeX specialize in layout design and are preferred for making a poster. Poster is exported for printing in PDF format.

Printing a Poster

Scientific posters are printed as a single sheet; the two choices of material are paper and polyester fibre. Matt paper becomes soggy when wet but colour does not run; glossy paper resembles a photographic paper; it is the preferred material. Polyester fabric is the best material and is waterproof, wrinkle resistant, fade resistant, and tear resistant. It is best to have the poster printed well before the travel date and carry it to the conference in a plastic tube that comes with shoulder straps. It is wise to carry a soft copy of the final version of the poster with you just in case the hard copy is damaged or lost.

ePosters

It is now a common practice to ask the poster submission in physical and electronic format. The soft version is displayed in kiosks in the conference complex or distributed to the attendees after the conference. The organizers often specify a templated format of the soft version which needs to be followed. Rules of display of text and graphics are similar for both the formats but the colours show better on the electronic display devices than on the printed media. A poster in electronic format is more effective in dissipating information than a physical one.

Defending a Poster

Most meeting organizers expect the presenters to be in attendance at a specified time to defend their work; this is an opportunity to interact with visitors and get first-hand feedback. The presentation format may be an open poster session, a poster symposium, or an oral presentation. It is important to know the expected audience during the presentation preparations, because that knowledge will influence how much time one needs to devote to discussing background information versus methodology, results, or conclusions. All research presentations are supposed to be persuasive in nature, whether introducing new ideas and technology or attempting to change existing standards. The main focus should concentrate on 'being true to the data' and allowing the results to support your conclusions and 'take-home messages'. Determining the knowledge and interest level of the expected audience will lead to a more 'targeted' presentation. A more specialized audience will require a more detailed presentation. This may facilitate making several 'take home points', whereas the goal for a general audience may be to make only the most important point.

Three presentations should be prepared for delivery at the poster: one for an observer with a general knowledge of the topic, a second for those with an advanced understanding, and a third for a group with diverse interests and understanding. The presenter should take the time to get introduced to each viewer on approach to the poster and use that as an opportunity to learn the attendee's position and knowledge of the topic. Presentations to viewers with a general knowledge should be less than 1 min, with 45 seconds given to describing the background, and 15 seconds dedicated to the take-home message. Details are generally lost on such viewers and should only be given if a specific question is asked. A poster should never be read to the viewer; it is referred to only if data presented in tables or graphs makes the results clearer. Presentations to viewers with advanced knowledge of the topic are the best and may last 5–10 min. Limiting the presentation to 3–5 min permits more time for discussion. Advanced viewers do not need background information and instead details of the methodology and results should be shared; the same 15-second are used for concluding remarks. If the results are clearly stated, the viewers will already know the take-home message. Advanced viewers are a treat and should be used as both learning sources and critics of the work. During these presentations, stop new visitors approaching the poster; they will benefit by eavesdropping on the current discussion, making a full presentation to them, unnecessary. Presentation to a small group at the poster combines the previous 2 presentations. This should be limited to 2–3 min, with single statement regarding the background and methods, heavy concentration on the results (using the poster graphics and tables), and a similar short conclusion.

Suggestions for Meeting Organizers

Organizers of a meeting can ease the task of the poster presenters. Instructions for the size of the posters should be circulated well before the meeting and should not be changed even if more than expected entries area received and the venue has limited space to fit those. The information about the type of display board, its location and lay out should be informed. All the necessary materials, like pins, tape, adhesive, etc., should be provided at the venue. However, presenters should carry their stock and not depend on the organizers. The conference attendees must be told what time the presenters will be available next to their own posters, so that there can be some interaction. Important attendees should make an advertised visit to discuss a few posters; recognition of a good work encourages better presentations in future. Locating coffee and food points in the poster display area is a smart way of attracting busy attendees (Fig. 13.9).

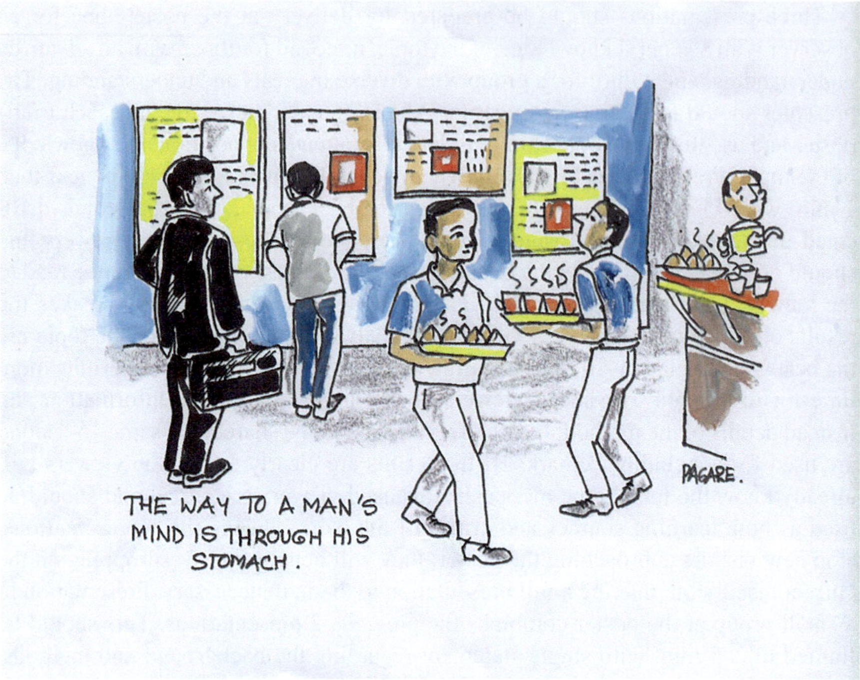
THE WAY TO A MAN'S MIND IS THROUGH HIS STOMACH.
PAGARE.

Fig. 13.9 Beverages and snacks in poster display zone increase footfalls

Further Reading

Abhishekh HA, Tandon N, Rangrajan S, Charaibeh A, Bonilla-Escobar FJ. Poster presentations: a presenting opportunity in conferences for medical students. Int J Med Students. 2014;2:35–6.

Briggs DJ. A practical guide to designing a poster for presentation. Nurs Stand. 2009;23(34):35–9.

Erren TC, Bourne PE. Ten simple rules for a good poster presentation. PLoS Comput Biol. 2007;3(5):e102. https://doi.org/10.1371/journal.pcbi.003010.

Ferreira JF, Patino CM. How to prepare and present a poster at a conference and communicate your research findings effectively. J Bras Pneumol. 2019;45(3):e2019016.

Goodhand JR, Giles CL, Wahed M, Irving PM, Langmead L, Rampton DS. Poster presentations at medical conferences: an effective way of disseminating research? Clin Med. 2011;11:138–4.

Hamilton CW. A stepwise approach to successful poster. Biostatistica. 2008;134:457–9.

Kaimal S, Thappa DM. The art and science of medical poster presentation. Indian J Dermatol Venereol Leprol. 2010;76:718–20.

Kobayashi KD, Perez K. A scientific poster is not a scientific article! 2015 Hawaii international conference on education (HICE) at: Honolulu, HI volume: pp. 1520–1530. 2015;

Persky AM. Scientific posters: a plea from a conference attendee. Am J Pharm Educ. 2016;80(10):162.

Singh MK. Preparing and presenting effective abstracts and posters in psychiatry. Acad Psychiatry. 2014, December;38(6):709–15. https://doi.org/10.1007/s40596-014-0190-z.

Thomas CE, Philip E, Bourne PE. Ten simple rules for a good poster presentation PLoS Comput Biol. 2007; 3: e102, p0777–8 www.ploscompbiol.or

An Approach to Podium and Webinar Presentations

14

Style is knowing who you are, what you want to say and not giving a damn — Gore Vidal

Contents

Supplementary Information The online version contains supplementary material available at [https://doi.org/10.1007/978-981-19-1816-2_14].

A. J. Thakur, *Tapping the Power of PowerPoint for Medical Posters and Presentations*, https://doi.org/10.1007/978-981-19-1816-2_14

How Does One Get to Speak in a Medical Meeting?

How does one get to speak in a medical meeting?; a submission is accepted or there is an invite. Each and every one involved in healthcare is required to give a presentation some time or other. PowerPoint and Keynote are popular apps for this purpose. Presentation skills are no longer optional but are essential for survival in the modern context. Scientific meetings offer opportunities for 3 types of talk.

Short Talk

A 8 to 10 minute talk is common for young presenters which follows acceptance of abstract of their research work. This talk has a standard format: IMRaD—Introduction, Material-method, Results, and Discussion. Quite often this type of presentation is part of a competition and it is necessary to follow whatever rules have been set by the organizers. The speakers in this category need guidance to make use of every moment of the short-allotted time. There is little scope to be careless and every slide must be well thought of and put together to tell the point under consideration.

Two longer versions are always by invitation and go to people with some standing in the speciality.

Medium Talk

The 20 to 30 minute lectures are usually educational, state of art, presentation of original research, a review of certain technique, or discussion of a clinical condition, etc. It could be stand-alone talk or part of a symposium with other speakers. There may be overlapping of topics in a session which should be found out at an early stage. Such talks to be successful should contain quality information and newest knowledge in the field. Speaker should make a list the impact points that he or she would like the audience to remember. The talk should be built around these nodes. There is usually time for questions.

Long Talk

The 50-minute talks are very special and are often orations, eponymous lectures, lifetime achievement talk, state-of-the-art talk, personal lecture, keynote lectures, etc. Talks in this category often contain anecdotes, personal comments, free advices, and messages. The speaker is senior and often distinguished in the field.

The speakers of these two categories are often experienced in presentation skills but still need guidance to rid of bad habits they might have picked up or an update on newer techniques of presentation.

Audience

Some guesswork on type of audience is important for any category of presentation. One needs to know the level of current knowledge of the audience on the topic of presentation. The level dictates the content of the presentation. A talk to residents would be different than to experienced consultants. Think of what the audience would like to know about the topic. It is equally important to decide what the speaker wants them to know about the research. And how much. Is the talk aimed at amusing the audience or to persuade? These thoughts should become the basis of the illustrations. What will be the size of the audience. A large 1500 capacity auditorium or a small room for 50 to 100 people. An interactive script is possible only with 30 to 40 persons.

What Are you Going to Say to this Audience

The creation of a presentation should not start in PowerPoint or Keynote but on a sheet of paper by writing down ideas, linking them to concepts and illustrations. This may be done in precise words that one wants to deliver or just a list of salient points. This has the same significance as preoperative planning in an orthopaedic operation. At the beginning one should clearly identify the subject of the talk by writing it down. Guiding thought should be what is the purpose of the presentation, what the audience is expected to do after hearing the talk, and what is the final message to achieve the ultimate objective. Audiences pay attention to new and interesting topics but are more interested in topics that are of practical use to them. 'what is in it for me' is a natural tendency that drives people to listen and take interest in a presentation. Occasionally a metaphor is used as the main heading. Metaphors carry some baggage of their own and a speaker should be careful not to choose one that may affect the tone of the presentation.

Providing too much information in a talk is counterproductive. A presentation should be used to raise awareness, provoke different ways of thinking, to inspire or motivate action about the main topic. Audiences tend to remember only up to 3 things even after a quality presentation. Important features should be told upfront.

A talk should have a beginning, middle, and the end. The hypothesis or the question should be explained at the beginning so the audience knows what the research is about. What was found doing the experiment should be told next with a reference to the research question. In the third part the audience should get the main message clearly and feel that they have gained new practical information that they may use in similar situations. Beginning of a talk can be effective if it has something novel, unexpected, challenging, personal, or humorous; good presentations often have one or two of these essentials. Novel topics always attract the audiences who have heard of it and have not had time to know more. A challenge always motivates the audiences to use their brains and pay attention. An unexpected quote, a question with a surprising answer shakes up an audience. Personal statements of anecdotal or academic interest would work for speakers with high professional standing; novice should stay clear of this approach. Humour and science just do not mix well. Response is often unpredictable and differs from audience to audience. A speaker should observe extreme caution in using humour; only those who have a knack of telling jokes to colleagues should attempt one; others should resist the temptation. Funny clips from YouTube are forbidden in scientific communications.

Talks should be prepared in advance. A scientific presentation is a performance and the outcome depends on the preparation. All physicians irrespective of years in the profession require preparation; when they do not, it shows. It is often obvious when a presentation was prepared on the way to the meeting or a day before. It appears sloppy, lacks the right words, and has abundant typos. Preparation should start at least 4 weeks prior to the event.

Gather Material for Emphasis

At this juncture a presenter should collect all the material that may be required to build the presentation. This may include existing slides, charts, graphics, statistics, quotations, photographs, logos, special drawings highlighting part of your theme, and videos. Visuals like these with explanatory text make a powerful communication tool.

Know the Details of day's Programme

In all the 3 categories of talk it is imperative to know where in the programme the lecture is planned and the speaking time assigned. Staying within the allotted time is good manners, and helps in maintaining the order of the conference; one speaker going over means others get less time and the question time is curtailed.

Time allotted to your talk also decides the size of the presentation. One needs to carefully decide the number of slides through practice and pacing and make sure there is time for questions and answers (Q & A). In a 10-minute talk first minute is spent in introduction and last two minutes are reserved for Q & A. Thus, in a 10-minute slot the practical talk time would only be 7 minutes.

Screen Dimensions and Types

Two prevalent aspect ratios of the projection screen are 4:3 and 16:9. The other technical information to have is the resolution of the projector: 1920 × 1080 (HD) and 1920 × 1200 are common values. The speaker should get in touch with the organizers and enquire the dimensions that will be used. The presentation apps offer these specifications. When starting a presentation correct value should be chosen. If the screen size and resolutions of the presentation and of the venue do not match, then the final projection will be suboptimal. It is also essential to know the projection system to be used. Will a digital projector be used or a LED wall will be used? The images on LED wall are far more brighter (1000 nits) than images from a digital projector (300 nits). When LED wall is available use of dark background for the slides do not irritate audience's eyes. When a digital light projector is in use light background slides are effective.

Limitations of the Conference Laptops and Projectors

Most conferences hire audiovisual equipment from vendors. The quality of laptops and projectors varies. Unless the organizers are tech savvy and specify their needs, the equipment company is at liberty to use available equipment that may be unsuitable for the venue and produce suboptimal projection. A presentation prepared on the newest computer with the latest version of PowerPoint or Keynote may not work when run on a 5-year-old computer operating on earlier version of the software. The laptop used in the conference room may have smaller memory than required and the presentation may hang up. Running videos in a conference becomes tricky because the software used on the conference computer and projector may not be able to handle a presentation. The image on the conference screen may appear faded due to mismatch in brightness of the projected image and ambient light. All these issues are beyond a speaker's control but by raising a concern about one's technical needs well before the conference may make the organizers aware and a solution could be found. The points made above allude to the importance of previewing the presentation in the speaker ready (preview) room at the conference. Large conferences do not allow a presenter to use personal computer; connecting and disconnecting a speaker's computer takes up valuable time; special adapters may be required; the software often do not match, and the battery habitually dies in the middle of the presentation.

Presentation Formats

Three formats ensure correctness in presentation. (1) Rhetoric format attributed to Aristotelean thinking, (2) Sherlock Holmes format, and (3) Columbo format.

Rhetoric format is popular and its authorship has been alluded to many. However, all quotation—researchers agree that the format is based on writings of Aristotle. It states: 'Tell them what you are going to tell them, tell them, then tell them what you told them'. The rhetoric format has been used extensively and is effective in all the three types of talks. Telling the audience what they are about to hear puts them in a receptive frame of mind for that topic and they stop guessing what is about to come. Telling them what has been told to is initiating the recapitulation mode and helps the audience to recall salient elements of the talk.

In Sherlock Holmes novels only on the last page one finds out who committed the murder; the rest of the novel is about the material, method, and discussion. If the last few pages of the novel are lost, then one does not know who did it. When the significant stuff is explained in the last few minutes of a talk, there is a possibility of audience missing out on the important points and lose out on the whole presentation due to speaker hurrying up to avoid running out of time, audience's dwindling interest in the proceedings, or other distractions.

Columbo is an American TV-detective. In first few minutes of each episode, the audience knows who committed the murder. The rest of the time is used to show how the detective zeros on the murderer. In a talk, audience attention is sharpest in first few minutes and it drops over a time. Once the main message is delivered in first instances, then little damage is done if the audience misses finer points of the result or discussion. In medical presentation, where time is at premium one should stay with Columbo format.

Start on PowerPoint

> When a man knows he is to speak in a fortnight it concentrates his mind wonderfully. – With apologies to Samuel Johnson

It has been said it is impossible for a Frenchman to speak with his hands in his pockets. The same sort of comment might be made about many of today's medical lecturers who find it almost impossible to communicate unless the lights are out and there is a chart, a graph, a list, a diagram, or picture on the screen. As and when one decides to deliver a lecture, may it be an 8-minute paper, a 25-minute symposium, or 50-minute oration, one should 'Think' what slide one needs and not what slides does one have for the lecture. Do not employ 'old Faithfulls'.

Why Do we Need Slides?

Slides are useful to reinforce a statement. Certain studies expound that recall rate improves if spoken words are followed by visuals, both graphic and text. A slide can supplement the spoken words; a graphic slide also is effective in this respect. It is a bit tedious to describe an unusual object but it is easy to show it on the screen and the add a few words to clarify the mute points. Slides can save considerable time when drawings form an essential part of the presentation; illustrations combined with clarifying text make best method to convey information accurately and rapidly. More specifically, in a scientific presentation, the slides should be used to put the work in perspective, to give distillation of the evidence for the case being presented, and to illustrate the results. The correct function of slides is to complement a talk in the same way that pictures enhance an advertisement and give a truthful, exact, apt, and striking description of the goods advertised. If a slide cannot be understood in 4 seconds, then it is an unacceptable slide; if people have to concentrate on working out the message of the slide they are not listening to the speaker. There are several misguided uses of a slide: it is used as reading Gizmo; entire paragraphs are projected and read aloud; as a filler slide between change of topics, during discussion time, or to hold audience's attention. Many speakers erroneously show slides of their own achievements, chance meeting with famous personalities, visits to foreign locations and even their natural history collections as a part of a scientific presentation.

An Acceptable Slide

A good slide can be appreciated by 7 adjectives. If any of these cannot be applied to a slide, it deserves to be junked.

Appropriate

Tables, graphs, and drawings produced in enough detail for journals (where they may be studied at leisure) are unsuitable for slides. The prominent points should be abstracted and where possible, presented as pictures, cartoons, or diagrams to produce an immediate effect. If words must be used, then only a précis should be given. The present practice of projecting entire sentences is deplorable.

Accurate

'However good your memory is, you should look up everything you quote'–Richard Asher. All the material put on the slide should be accurate. The spellings and grammar must be checked several times manually and by using the computer spelling program. This is true if someone else is preparing the slides for the presentation. Errors are not always accidental, nor are they restricted to text. When drawing a graph, for example, it is possible to show bias to the point of dishonesty if drawn with vertical axis showing 40% at the bottom and 45% at the top, instead of 0 and 100% (Fig. 14.1).

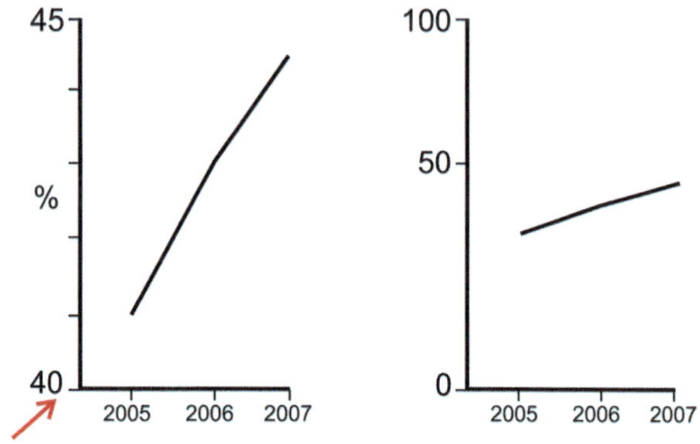

Fig. 14.1 I do not mind lying but I hate inaccuracy-Samuel Butler

Legible

Never use full stops—they disturb the visual flow of type—and sparingly use other punctuation marks. Secondly, choose capital letters and lower case consistently. Use Spaces between letters, words, and lines with care. Use sans serif typeface. In summary slides, asterisk or dots are more eye-catching than numbers viz. 1, 2, 3, etc. in propounding the key points. Quite apart from the visual effect, numbers indicate a diminishing order of importance which is not always what one wishes to convey.

Make full use of available space. It is of vital importance that only a limited volume of information should appear on each slide. Presenter is the only person who can design slides with minimum text on the slide. Medical art department or a computer technician cannot design such a slide for presentation.

Comprehensible

How often one hears a speaker comment apologetically, 'this slide may look rather complicated' This is an understatement and only signifies that the speaker has not taken the time and trouble to simplify it. Complicated formulae and detailed experimental methods have no place on slides (Fig. 14.2). They need only to be mentioned by the speaker, and those who want the details can be referred to a published work. Abbreviations, though tempting, should be used with care—particularly if the audience is international. Certain standard ones have been published, but is sensible to explain any other that you may use.

Well Executed

This is closely related to legibility. It should be remembered that an ugly layout suggests an ugly product (Fig. 14.3). Slides should be well balanced and, where possible, designed to be shown horizontally rather than vertically as there are surprisingly few lecture halls in which the screen does not cut off one end of a vertical slide.

Fig. 14.2 Incomprehensible. Suitable for publication but not for a slide presentation

$$
\begin{gathered}
var(S)=1\{n(n-1)(2n+5)-\varepsilon\tau(t-1)(2T+5)-\mu(\mu-1)(2\mu+5)\} \\
1\{9\ \mu(\eta-1)(\eta-2)[\varepsilon\tau(\tau-1)(\tau-2)\}\{\varepsilon\mu(\mu-1)(\mu-2)\} \\
+2\eta(\eta-1)\{\varepsilon\tau(\tau-1)\}\{\varepsilon\upsilon(\upsilon-1)\theta+2\sigma(\sigma-1)(\delta-2)\}(\omega+\varepsilon+\rho)(\tau+\Psi+\gamma) \\
1\{8\ \delta(\eta-\phi)(\eta-5)[\theta\tau(\omega\tau-1)(\gamma\tau-2)\}\{\varepsilon\mu(\mu-1)(\mu-2)\} \\
+2\varpi(\eta-1)\{\xi\varepsilon\tau(\tau-1)\}\{\varepsilon\chi\upsilon(\upsilon-1)\theta+2\varpi\sigma(\sigma-1)(\delta-2)\}(\omega\nu+\varepsilon+\rho)(\tau+\Psi+\gamma)
\end{gathered}
$$

Fig. 14.3 'Ill-executed and inaccurate. Proportions wrong, capital letters scattered through, words misspelled, and spacing inconsistent

PLAIN RADIOLOGY - 50 paTients

8 "Stenosis sPINALE" Cases proved at surgery

- Measurement and "Ration Analysis" failed to isolate Stenosis Cases

Always write horizontally when anointing the vertical axis of a graph. Never use a graph paper as a background because the lines confuse and distract. Use of colour has a significant overall effect. We are brought up to relate a colour to certain circumstances, for example, that red implies danger or heat, green safety, and blue peace or cold. Some find the blue and white restful; some would describe it is soporific. A most useful colour is white, not only in its own right but also to point or balance other colours.

Interesting

You cannot bore people into appreciating your research. If your slides are dull, inaccurate, badly made, and illegible, your audience will either go to sleep or leave the hall. When presenting with 50 or more other papers at a research meeting where each one of the audience has his own axe to grind a presenter needs to go an extra mile to create interesting slides (Fig. 14.4). 'A person who desires to make an impression must stand out in some way from the masses'-Hopkins.

Memorable

There are a few memorable slides. We all know which they are—we remember them (Fig. 14.5).

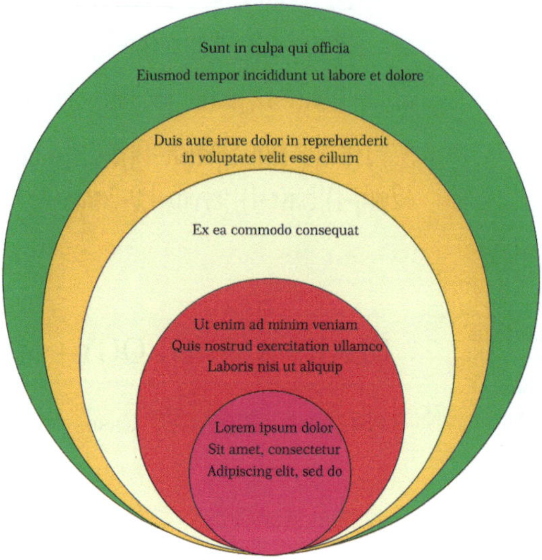

Fig. 14.4 Use of colour, novel shape, and unusual layout makes it an interesting slide

Fig. 14.5 Memorable slides do not need description; they are memorable

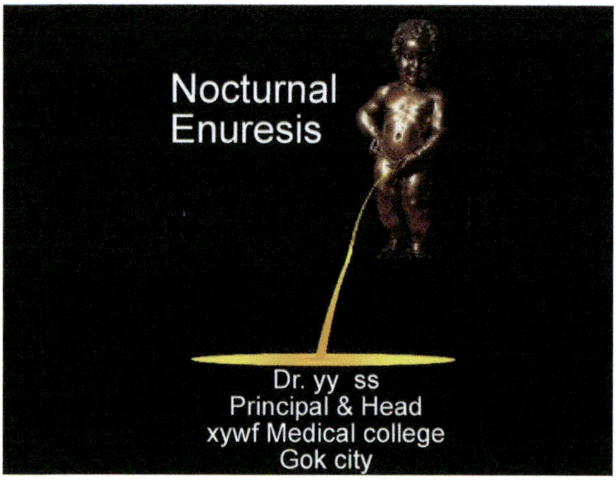

Slide Design

Most templates stink. Horribly. Abhor templates as they add clutter and distract from visual impact of a slide; they are overused and are cliché. It is best to use a blank slide and create a design.

Design of a slide for scientific presentation is about simplicity and not about decoration. Every element should have a positive impact on the message. Any component that is irrelevant to the topic harms learning and eliminating unwanted material improves it. Some institutes have templates that the staff is expected to use it during their presentations. Such templates have distracting unconnected material. A way to get out of this predicament is to prepare a colour palette based on institutional colours and use the combination for the background and text.

Background, Typeface Combination, and Colour Scheme

Essential features of a slide are background, typeface, and colour scheme. One needs to make a choice on all these elements at the beginning and stay with it throughout the presentation. A consistent look projects a positive image of the presenter and of the research being presented. As a variety one may change one of these features to indicate change of topic during the presentation. However, this trick should not be overdone.

Number of slides required for a presentation is dependent on the presenter. It is difficult to put down a scale like so many slides for a 10-minute talk and is impossible to do so for longer versions. In general, every slide should serve a purpose and take the presentation forward. A slide that fails to add value should be discarded, fewer the better. Not a single slide in the presentation should be superfluous, ever.

Use of animation should be with a purpose and not as a fancy trick. PowerPoint and Keynote offer a large number of elaborate animations but one should choose simple ones for a specific purpose. As novelty wears out quickly the audience gets tired of fancy animations. Animation slows down the speed of presentation; when presentation time is limited animations should be avoided.

Language and Spell Check

Speaking and writing in a language correctly is an attitude. It has to be developed by dedication and practice. When this attitude is lacking not only English, any language is spoken badly. English is the universal language of science and medicine. Non-native English speakers often want to cover up their shortcomings by saying it is not their mother tongue. If one wants to excel, good command over the language of presentation is important.

Spelling checkers are essential tools for presentation and must always be used. They are not full-proof. Manual spelling check is also necessary to overcome some peculiarities of the English spellings.

Contents of a Slide

A slide text should be an indicator of what one is saying and should not get repeated. At any instance, the slide should show only one line on what is being talked. Occasional use of two-bullet slide is fine; repeated use of multiple bullets is amateurish. When next 3 to 4 points are displayed, the audience quickly reads them and waits to catch up rather than listen to the narration. The presentation sequence should be to display one point on the slide and elaborate; sequence may also be reversed. Audience can recall a full sentence headline better than a word or phrase.

Large paragraphs of a text should not be projected; audience's attention is split between listening and reading. Audience reads the matter quicker than the speaker can deliver. Should a big text slide be unavoidable, progressive disclosure helps. If one needs a prompt card, 'presenter view' should be used (Fig. 14.6). In this optional view, a speaker can see the slide that is being projected, the next slide to come in and read out the commentary which is visible only to him. The speaker should always face the audience even while reading the projected text.

Less is more—Keep a slide sparsely populated. One image with short descriptive embedded text is most effective format for visual communication.

Images in a Slide

The purpose of illustration is to telegraph the message to the reader — Ogilvy.

One of the surveys on use of presentation apps concluded: when just text is displayed audience assimilation is 7%, with only oral input it is 38%, and with visual aids it is 55%. A combination of three, oral statement and an illustration with embedded text makes a substantial impact on the audience. However, the image on the screen must be relevant to the subject; it should be instantly evident why the audience is looking at it and it should reinforce the spoken words; addition of an explanatory text enhances the impact. Images may be photographs, charts, or drawings. When the charts or figures are from separate sources, to look more consistent in the presentations they may be drawn again using programs like CorelDraw or

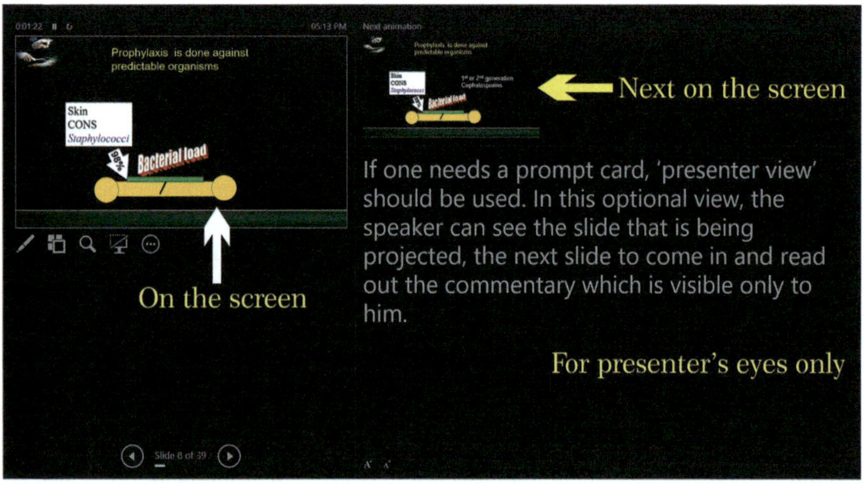

Fig. 14.6 The presenter view is speaker's discreet prompt card

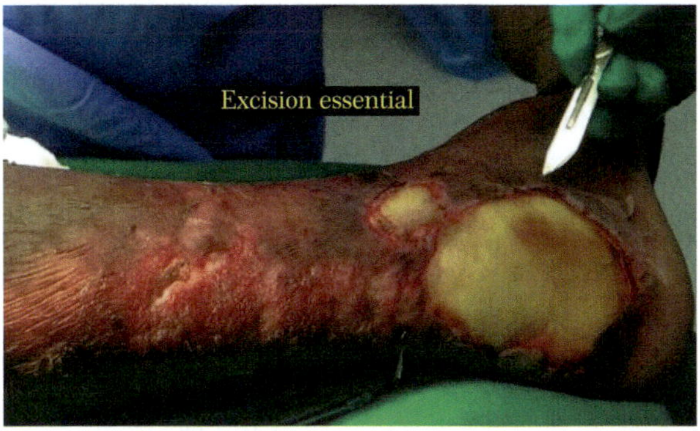

Fig. 14.7 'Good quality photographs should fill the whole slide'

Affinity Designer. Two popular ways of using images is to make a statement and show the supportive image or show an image first and follow it by narration. This is like a Waltz; sometimes the speaker leads, sometimes the slide leads. Every photo in a presentation should be of high quality. A photo should fill the whole slide. A text over a photo should be easily read; adding a screen box in the background of the text assures readability (Fig. 14.7). Shapes with rounded corners make a better impact. Photos downloaded from web pixilate when projected and may not be used.

Use of Transition and Animation

PowerPoint and Keynote offer a wide variety of slide transitions and animations. These should be used sparingly in a scientific presentation (Video 14.1). Default slide transition is most satisfactory but other sequences may be used occasionally to stress a point or two. It is recommended to use animation in deploying computer generated arrows and altogether avoid use of laser or wooden pointers. A 'dynamic' computer generated arrow is more effective when it 'appears' on a click than a 'static' arrow which appears with the slide. Apart from this basic animation there are tens of fancy ones which should only be used occasionally, when serving a purpose, and not to show-off computer skills.

Edit Ruthlessly when Finished; Use Slide Sorter

'Perfection is achieved, not when there is nothing more to add, but when there is nothing left to take away'. Antoine De Saint-Exupery; perfection is elusive but 'we can achieve excellence only through pursuit of perfection' alluded to Maurice E Müller.

After the creation of a presentation is complete, it is time to edit, ruthlessly. If something is unappealing, distracting, or confusing, it must be deleted; chances are the overall presentation will be the better. This is best done in 'Slide sorter' or 'light table' view. In these views, it is easy to capture configuration of the entire presentation. One sees several slides at a glance and can identify the logical flow of the presentation and if needed make multiple changes on the go. A complicated slide is promptly identified in this view which then can be broken down into two or three simple ones. Similarly, unnecessary slides can be quickly deleted to increase visual clarity and improve communication.

Rehearse

The presentation and speaker should work in tandem; slides should complement the talk and talk should be compatible with the slides; it is matter of timing. Timing comes with practice; rehearsing the talk is the key to a good presentation. A well-rehearsed speaker does not need to read from the slides, or even look at them. Reading the script loudly several times helps in the final delivery. Practice is the road to perfection. Multiple rehearsals elevate an average presentation to a respectable one. Honest feedback may be received from friendly critics like family, friends, partners, colleagues, and children. Use of video or audio recording is a fine tool for practice and self-analysis. The adage, 'if you fail to prepare, you are prepared to fail', is worth remembering (Video 14.2).

Before the Presentation Day

Day, date, and time are important and should be double checked. Check the venue too; Mayo Clinic is in Rochester; there are 19 Rochester towns in America and 3 in the United Kingdom. A presentation should be carried to the meeting on two storage devices, kept in two different places in the luggage and an additional copy in the cloud. Cue cards are traditional aide memoires and should be readied before the travel.

On the Presentation Day

During the Presentation

Dressing well is a form of good manners — Tom Ford.

A speaker should dress-up for a scientific talk. Avoid dressing like a technician in T-shirt, shorts, baseball cap worn other way round and chappals; learned audience of a medical meeting deserves a minimum of social grace. In India and other hot countries smart shirts and ties are a safe passport to respectability. Winter meetings in north India require warm suits; dark-coloured ones are preferred choices. Very fancy and flashy neckties may be avoided. Well-kept beard or clean-shaven gentlemen always score over the unshaven who flaunt stubs proclaiming their lazy and careless attitude. Avoid wearing things that will divert the audience's attention away from the talk. Shoes and socks will complete the list; avoid white socks as they show when one sits on the dais as a faculty. Women speakers should not dress to kill (Fig. 14.8). Avoid flashy accessories and flower bouquets in hair. Jewellery should be sober.

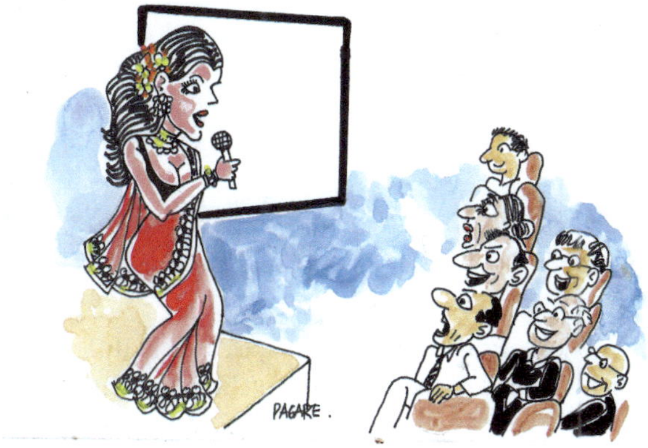

Fig. 14.8 '*You* are the focus, no matter how interesting your slides are'

A Speaker should arrive early and submit the presentation in the speaker ready or preview room. Presentation should run smoothly on the available computers; videos require special attention. Lavaliere microphone allows freedom to move about without dropping the voice; a request for one should be made in the preview room. A request for a step-up platform for a short statured presenter should be made in the preview room. When in good time a presenter should try and sit in on a talk in the same room early in the day to get a feel for the acoustics and the audiovisual facilities. The presenter should be in the room a few minutes early than the appointed hour and get acquainted with audiovisual arrangements, the hall managers, and the chairperson. Next, the projectionist should be explained the plan for the slides and the arrangements for dimming the lights. Presenter view, if needed, should be requested. This is the time to make sure the stepping up platform is available for a short statured speaker. The presenter should occupy a seat reserved for faculty near the stage. When called out, speaker should approach the lectern unhurriedly and take stock of the available audiovisual gadgets and adjust the microphone, lavalier or fixed; cue cards or text section of the presenter view is adjusted to comfort. The pointer is a hazard. Use of a wooden pointer like a magician's wand to ward off the evil spirits is unbecoming in scientific meeting. Unless the speaker needs to draw attention to some object, laser pointer may not be switched on; constantly switched on and pointed at the screen, a laser beam creates a 'pointer doodle', a distracting aimless movement of laser beam on the screen during the talk (Fig. 14.9). Laser or wooden pointer should altogether be dispensed with by pre-planning the use of computer generated block arrows for accuracy and time saving (see page). Several meetings have a digital timer for the speaker; a personal timepiece with large luminous hands placed on the lectern is an alternative. Loudly rehearsing the talk several times before the event also helps in maintaining the time limits. Presenter should set the stopwatch and start the talk with appropriate opening.

Opening sentences should be delivered with lights on, without referring to the notes, and establishing eye contacts with the audience. Lights may be dimmed after the introductory statements. Use of microphone needs to be learnt. Holding a

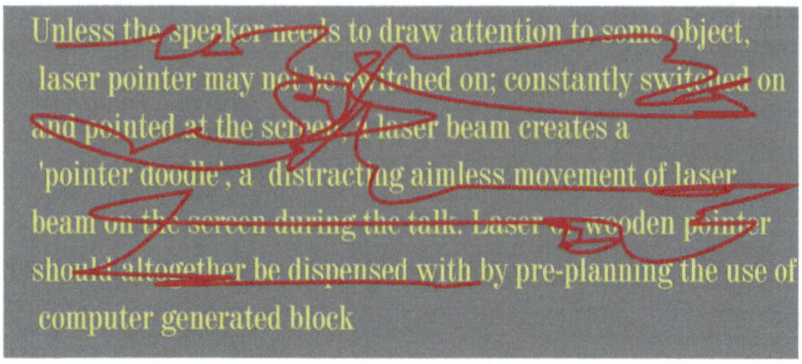

Fig. 14.9 A laser doodle can be very distracting

microphone in the hand while speaking is different from speaking into a microphone attached to the lectern. Lavaliere mike is a pleasure and allows unsurpassed freedom of movement to the speaker. A word on voice production is not out of place. Even with a microphone, a presenter should speak up front and address the back row of the hall. Only then everyone in the hall will hear the talk. The end of a sentence must not be dropped but said loudly. A sentence is valueless unless it is heard in the last row. Speaking on the move may be avoided. One topic ended, presenter should take a breath and organize the thoughts before starting again; such a break adds vigour to the voice and the presentation. The microphones may misbehave. When it goes dead in the middle of the talk, the presenter should move close to the seated audience and continue addressing the last row of the room. Once the technician is able to re-establish the sound system, microphone may be used again. Sound distortions such as popping noises are caused when the microphone is held too close to the mouth. Moving the microphone farther away and turning the head a bit helps. A wireless microphone also needs to be moved to another location. In both the situations, increasing the distance settles the issue. A high pitched hissing sound indicates that two or three microphones are switched on simultaneously. Shutting down the unused ones solves the problem. A talk should be delivered at a rate that sounds slow to the speaker; audience does not perceive it so. Similarly, more emphasis than normal by a speaker is not sensed as too theatrical by the audience. Suitable hand and facial gestures should be used to project the presenter's enthusiasm. A good speaker should not 'speak' to the slides by turning his back to the audience while reading the material on the screen. One should never read from the slides. A talk should be concluded forcefully and finished by thanking the audience for attention. Avoid 'Thank you' slide. While waiting for the questions speaker should bring back the title slide. Initiating questions on the talk is chair's prerogative and a speaker may not encroach.

In an event of running out of time, a presenter should not panic, but take dignified action by using navigational keyboard shortcuts and reach concluding slides without audience realizing the slip, wrap up the performance in style, and continue grabbing audience's attention. Disaster planning includes carrying a PDF version of the presentation in a smart phone to serve as a prompt card should there be equipment failure or power outage. Presentation is no longer an option but an essential skill for anyone who wants to achieve a position in medical profession.

After the Presentation

Handouts

Printing the slides as handouts does not serve any purpose because the text on the slides is cryptic in nature and one needs the speaker's help to make sense out of it. Handouts should be written separately with details not covered in the oral presentation. The handouts should be passed out after the talk; if given before, audience gets busy reading it and does not pay attention. Distribution of a PDF by email is the current trend.

Question Time

Who questions much, shall learn much, and retain much — Francis Bacon

Meeting organizers value question-and-answer time and allot 17–20% of the talk time for the audience participation. Almost all presentations are followed by question-and-answer session. The real adrenaline flows during this session because of its uncertain nature. Loaded questions may fly-in from unexpected directions and may 'get' the presenter. A speaker is usually well informed about the presented material than anyone else in the meeting. This is a position of strength and should boost presenter's confidence. It is not knowing all the answers but anticipating all the questions that gives the confidence to a speaker. Question time like rest of the presentation requires preparation. All the possible questions should be noted and apt answers prepared. Use of additional slides on methodology, technique, statistics to reinforce the planned answer creates a positive impression; such slides may be prepared and added to the presentation. A mock question-answer session with colleagues helps in identifying the questions and in fine tuning the answers.

See-hear compatibility principle of presentation implies prevalence of compatibility between what the audience sees on the screen and what audience hears; when such agreeableness exists, the audience retains almost all of the presented material. However, during question time one often sees slides with a thank-you note, acknowledgements, a slide appealing to ask questions, a list of references, a combination of these or PowerPoint's default black screen announcing end of the slide show. Some organizers use this time to display administrative notices or even a sponsored message. These visuals are not compatible with the question session. The audience members are less likely to learn the answers to the questions being asked unless see-hear compatibility is maintained throughout the session. To create a compatible milieu a presenter should first note down the numbers of important slides. When answering the question, the relevant slide should be recalled to create see-hear compatibility. If such a slide does not exist, a white blank slide should be shown. This brings additional brightness on the lectern; the presenter comes in focus; the audience takes in every spoken word. After the question has been answered the title slide

Fig. 14.10 Keyboard shortcuts for random slide selection during a presentation

Keyboard short cuts to navigate between the slides
Work for PC and Mac
In slide show view

Press 1	+ enter	to display the first slide
Press 22	+ enter	to display slide number 22
Press slide number	+ enter	to display desired slide
Press W	+ enter	to display white screen
Press B	+ enter	to display black screen

should be projected again. The speaker himself should use the keyboard shortcuts to navigate between the slides and bring on the most compatible slide (Fig. 14.10). Practice makes this interchange a seamless affair.

A typical talk includes a question-and-answer time. As the chairperson invites questions from the floor, no one wants to face dead silence! Often the first question is slow to come by and valuable time is lost. A useful strategy is to make a suggestion in final phase of the talk: 'in next couple of minutes, I will conclude and answer all the questions that you may have; so start thinking about you questions now'. Such a phrase stimulates the audience to think and they are ready to field a question at the first chance. A colleague may be tasked to ask the first question as soon as the opportunity arises; this saves time; questions subsequently flow in steady stream. A colleague may also be coached to ask such a question that helps to present additional material which due to time constraints was not included. A speaker should repeat a question for 3 reasons: It gives time to think; some members of the audience may not have heard the question. Repeating a question presents an opportunity for clarification if the question was heard incorrectly.

The answer should be short and to the point; it should not be a mini-lecture. Whenever possible, a question should be rephrased to link up with suitable slide in the presentation. A speaker should develop a finesse to take a question on the fly and shape it into an appropriate inquiry or point for which an answer is ready (Fig. 14.11). A question also may be rephrased in a roundabout way to state what the speaker would have liked to say. It is unwise to say that a question is bad or has already been addressed. Similarly belittling a question or its originator is bad policy. It may hurt the speaker in several ways. Each person who asks a question should be thanked regardless of the content of the question. Always be polite and respectful to the audience.

It is not possible to know all the answers; face-saving answers could be, 'interesting, I will look into that or 'that is a good point, let's discuss it afterwards'. A smart move is to divert the question to a senior colleague. It is also perfectly acceptable to say that one does not know the answer. Some attendees ask multiple questions. A speaker should answer one or two of those questions and then recognize other attendees to ask a question. Occasionally a questioner turns aggressive and wants to initiate an argument. The situation could be defused by using the aphorism, 'We agree to disagree on this point'; 'let us take other questions now and we may

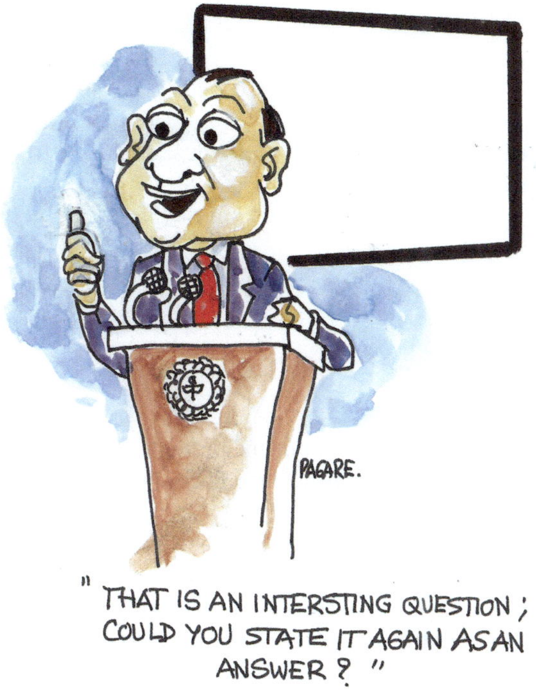
PAGARE.
"THAT IS AN INTERSTING QUESTION;
COULD YOU STATE IT AGAIN AS AN
ANSWER?"

Fig. 14.11 A clever speaker may contort a question to his advantage

continue to discuss this over a cup of tea'. Question time is useful if one wants to write up research for a journal. It identifies lacunae in the presented analysis and hints to the areas that were poorly understood by the audience.

Each presenter should have an individual question time. Each one gets a fair share if the questions are asked immediately after the talk. Many times, a chairperson decides to take all the questions at the end of the session (Fig. 14.12). This practice is unfair to the presenters because in a group, a few of the presenters do not get any questions while some get a handful. It is also too much to expect of the audience to remember all the questions that they would have liked to ask, if given a chance just after each talk. A presenter who would like a compartmentalized question-answer session should make it known to the chairperson before the start of the session.

Ten high-profile orthopaedic surgeons who are also sought-after speakers participated in a 2021-survey on methods to prepare for the question time. They approved of dry-runs to practice questions-answers with professional colleagues. Most of them reserved making of additional slides for longer formats of the presentation. All were aware of the keyboard shortcuts to navigate through the slides and considered the tactic a face-saving move when running out of time which they meticulously try to avoid. All of them value question time and prefer specific

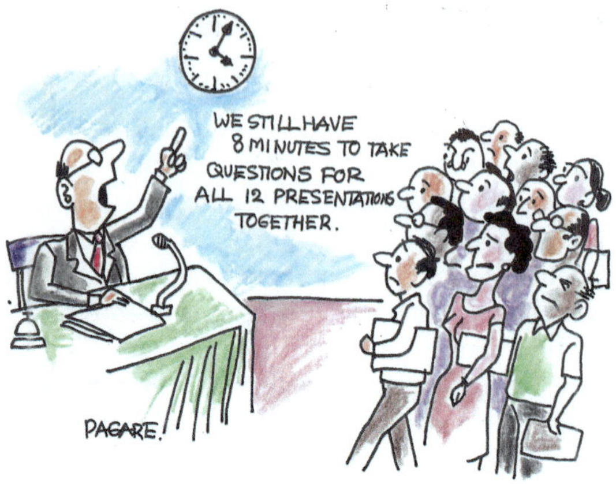
WE STILL HAVE
8 MINUTES TO TAKE
QUESTIONS FOR
ALL 12 PRESENTATIONS
TOGETHER.
PAGARE

Fig. 14.12 Each speaker deserves separate question time

questions on the subject of the presentation; all dislike long winding monologues and multiple questions by a member of the audience.

Audience and Question Time

> Light travels faster than sound. This is why some people appear bright until you hear them speak — Alan Dundes

Asking questions in a scientific meeting is a responsibility (Fig. 14.13). It should be done with decorum. The chair's permission should be sought before fielding a question. Each person asking a question should state name and place he or she comes from. It is very civil to complement a speaker before asking the question but this nicety consumes valuable time and may be skipped or used only in the shortest format. A question may be asked seeking clarification, analysis, comparison, or relationship of the topic under discussion. One should state the question clearly and briefly; a question should never be asked in an aggressive manner. Arguments should be shunned; deep disagreements should be sorted out after the session, over a cup of tea and end in smoking peace pipe. Question time should not be taken as an opportunity to make a long statement on a similar research conducted by the questioner or his associates. Multiple questions from one individual robs others of an opportunity to ask questions. Approaching a speaker after a lecture to ask a question is often rewarding as he is more relaxed while answering.

Chairperson of a Meeting

> An audience always appreciates a firm chairperson. Indeed, the comparative qualities of a good chairperson have been described as "tough, tougher, and toughest" — Anonymous

Why are you asking a question?

Introspection tool for a prospective questioner

Seeking soulful answers to these questions will help others in the conference

Do you want clarification on something not well presented in the lecture

Do you think your question will add value to the talk

Do you want to ask a question to help the presenter who is your friend

Do you want to ask the question to pull down the presenter whom you hate

Do you want the presenter to repeat the matter even though it was clearly presented earlier

Do you want to ask a question because you had arrived late, fallen asleep, or looking at someone cute when the matter was presented and you missed

Your know the answer; do you still want to ask and test the presenter

Do you want to ask the question even though it is not related to the presented topic

Do you want to know a minute insignificant detail just for the sake of perfection

Do you want to make a statement on some thing related to the topic

Do you want to start a monologue under the guise of asking a question on entirely unrelated topic

Do you want to show-off your knowledge of the topic by asking a question

Do you want to ask a question to establish that you are a compulsive obsessive questioner

Do you want to ask a question because you think it is a requirement to get attendance certificate

Fig. 14.13 'Asking a question is often not "just" asking a question; it sometimes has a deeper meaning' — Jim A Reekers

Meeting organizers need a chairperson to run the show. In him the organizers choose a person to do their bidding of running a part of the meeting on schedule, seamlessly, and with decorum. They often choose a few experienced people from the list of attendees; some attendees perceive it as an honour and solicit chairpersonships. Either way it is a responsibility. After accepting the invitation, one should ask for a copy of the meeting's programme and details of the earmarked session. This helps the prospective chairperson to manage his or her time during the entire meeting. Next the soon-to-be chairperson should obtain a copy of the abstract of the papers to be presented in the designated session and study them. It is essential for a potential chairperson to formulate a few questions on each topic to be presented in that session. A chairperson must ask a question if none are forthcoming from the audience. An accomplished chairperson learns proper pronunciations of the speakers' names, e.g. Valéry Giscard d'Estaing. On the day of the session a chairperson should dress maturely to suit the importance of the meeting. Chairperson should arrive early in the specified room and should acquaint himself with audiovisual people and with the organizer's mid-level representatives in-charge. If the timekeeping mechanism is run by the audio-visual team (AV Team), then they should be instructed to start the clock only after the speaker starts talking and not on arrival at the lectern; this ensures that a speaker is not shortchanged for time. Light dimming mechanisms should be checked as total darkness in a room is

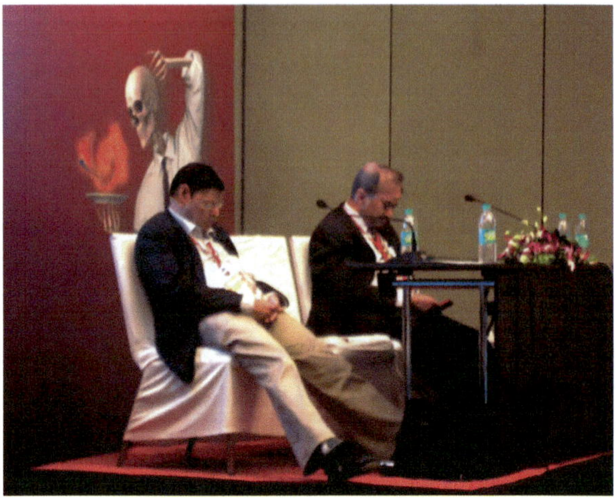

Fig. 14.14 Chairing a session is a responsibility and not a place to relax or catch nine winks

not necessary; modern projectors are effective in a partially lit room; some ambient light is desirable.

A chairperson should meet the speakers as they arrive and make them at ease. Starting the proceedings in time is chairperson's responsibility. Each topic should be announced with a personal touch and not merely read out in monotone. Throughout the session a chairperson should be attentive, not pour over a smartphone or worse, doze off; snoring chairperson is a big embarrassment (Fig. 14.14). It is the duty of the chairperson to maintain speaking time for each and every presenter. Eminent speakers may try to hoodwink the time restrictions and go well beyond; such people need a tough chairperson. Role of a chairperson is secondary to that of the speaker; it should not be reversed. A chairperson should lead question-and-answer time; open it, regulate the numbers, and close it when it is time. In a session that has several speakers on similar topics it is best not to club the question times in one because this often denies the speakers of their chance to individually defend respective presentations. A chairperson should ensure that there is an equal opportunity for all the attendees to ask questions and prevent a person from fielding serial questions (Video 14.3). If no questions are forthcoming, then a chairman should ask one to keep the ball rolling. Some questioners take the opportunity to start their own monologue under the guise of asking questions; such people need a tough chairperson. When the time is over, the chairperson may quickly summarize the proceedings, thank the speakers and the audience and declare the session as closed. A competent chairperson can make a session lively and take it to a higher level.

Webinars

I learned far more than I was expecting — Helena Leyva-Sanchez

Webinars allow learners time to "breathe" in between sessions—to rethink, reflect and an opportunity for application — Anonymous

Webinars became popular in 2020 due to restrictions on physical meetings during Covid-19 pandemic. The basic tenets of presentation on a webinar are same as the one for podium presentation. However, each speaker is on his own without any guidelines for the meetings. The speaker himself has to make all the technical arrangements for the participation. Most people use their laptop or desktop to participate.

Timings

Like all physical meetings precise timings should be followed. This is significant because physical distance has no relevance in webinars. Audience may be located in several time zones in different parts of the world.

Dress

Although the presenters are in the comfort zones of their homes, they are in a virtual public place as they are being seen by people all across the world. Several speakers dress up casually since they are speaking from their home. This is disrespectful to the audience. It really does not matter where the presenter is located, at home or hospital, he or she should dress up as if speaking from a conference hall. If the talk is official, then the speaker should appear like a person on official work and not one on a holiday. A well-groomed appearance is always more impressive than a casual look with unshaven and unkept hair. Webinar audience expects a speaker to be properly dressed.

Background

In a webinar, background matters (Fig. 14.15). Speaking from home, one has little control over what is seen behind the presenter. This should be controlled by applying technology. Any picture file in jpeg or png format can be adopted as a virtual background in a webinar. Distracting background slides showing trans-harbour bridges, Goan beaches, or Himalayan mountains should be avoided (Fig. 14.16).

A pastel coloured plain background slide is a pleasant and non-distracting alternative choice. A logo or the conference title in the background is welcome because it serves as an identification tag. Any single PowerPoint and Keynote slide can be exported to jpeg or png format and used as a background in a webinar.

Camera Position

Most webinar presenters use laptop or desktop cameras to join in. The camera should be at the speaker's eye level. The camera may be adjusted to show the

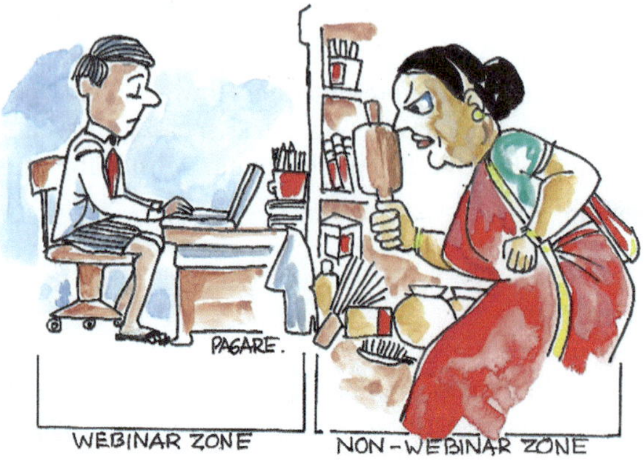

Fig. 14.15 Webinar offers unrestricted home comforts to a keynote speaker

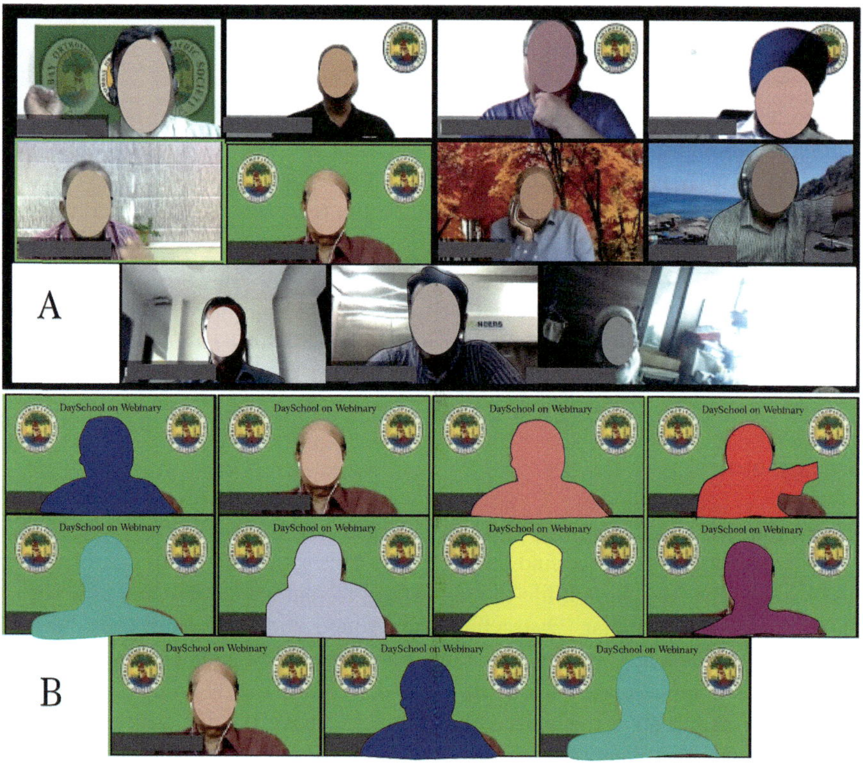

Fig. 14.16 Distracting backgrounds. (**a**) Variegated and varicoloured background in each window gives this montage an appearance of a casual chat group. (**b**) Uniform background with institutional logo metamorphoses this motely group to an official seminar faculty

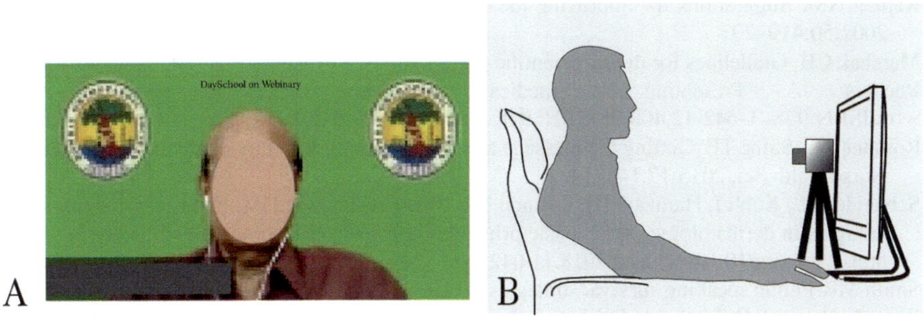

Fig. 14.17 Camera set-up for webinar. (**a**) The speaker's image should appear at the junction of upper one-third and lower two-third in the centre of the screen. (**b**) Use of a professional camera for webinar ensures a superior image composition; the screen may be used as a teleprompter

speaker's image in the centre of the screen leaving some room above the head (Fig. 14.17). Use of a head phone, wired or wireless is recommended for clarity of transmission and to cut off the extraneous sounds. The presenter should look into the camera and speak. A frequent speaker on webinar should invest in a quality web camera with a tripod stand. It may be placed in front of the computer screen. The computer screen then can serve as a teleprompter.

Organization of an International Webinar

Different time zones are a matter of consideration in international webinars. When time zones are cordial for all concerned, a live webinar is practical. When time zones are difficult or the event is of importance, prerecorded presentation is a practical choice. This precludes disruptions due to connectivity problems and video outages. At the appointed time the recording of the presentation is played flawlessly. The presenter then joins live for a question-answer session thus reducing the risk of interruptions and failures.

Further Reading

Evans M. The use of slides in teaching-a practical guide. Med Educ. 1981;15:186–91.

Grech V. WASP (write a scientific paper): optimisation of PowerPoint presentations and skills. Early Hum Dev. 2018;125:53–6.

Ferreira JF, Patino CM. How to prepare and present a poster at a conference and communicate your research findings effectively. J Bras Pneumol. 2019;45(3):e2019016.

Falcone JL. After the applause: how to use PowerPoint effectively during the question and answer portion of a presentation. Am Surg. 2013;79:332–4.

Greenhalgh T. Preparing and delivering a 10-minute presentation at a scientific meeting. Paediatr Respir Rev. 2011; https://doi.org/10.1016/j.prrv.2011.01.01.

Jones AM. The use and abuse of PowerPoint in teaching and learning in the life sciences: a personal overview. Biosci Educ. 2003;2(1):1–13. https://doi.org/10.3108/beej.2003.0200000.

Kaplan NM. Suggestions for improving the effectiveness of oral presentations. J Investig Med. 2002;50:419–20.

Marchak CB. Guidelines for digital scientific presentations. J Prosthet Dent. 2002;88:649–53.

Reekers JA. Presenting at medical meetings. Heidelberg: Springer. 2010; e-ISBN:978–3–642-12,408-2; ISBN: 978–3–642-12,407-5 2010.

Rossiter RC, Stone TE. Getting the message across: Delivering a quality conference presentation. Nurs Health Sci. 2015;17:145–14.

Schneider SL, Kohli I, Hamzavi IH, Council ML, Rossi AM, Ozog DM. Emerging imaging technologies in dermatology: part I: basic principles. J Am Acad Dermatol. 2019;80(4):1114–20. https://doi.org/10.1016/j.jaad.2018.11.042.

Smith MF. Public speaking survival strategies. J Emerg Nurs. 2000;26:166–8.

Watts E, Peacock O, Liyanage S, Elsey E, Lund J. Presentation skills amongst surgical trainees at a national conference: an observational study. J R Soc Med. 2012;3:30. https://doi.org/10.1258/shorts.2011.011134.

Unteregger F, Mayer P. Medical lectures upgraded: 11 hacks from comedy. GMS J Med Educ. 2019;36(3):Doc23. ISSN 2366–5017

Audiovisual Planning for a Large Medical Conference

15

'The magic to a great meeting is all of the work that's done beforehand' — *Bill Russell*

Contents

Audiovisual arrangements in a conference have the power to make or break a conference. The purpose of a meeting is to communicate information to peers and colleagues which needs good audiovisual arrangements. Although the gaffes of the mounted-slide era like projecting images upside down have disappeared with change of technology, newer glitches have appeared. Presentations made in the Keynote program will not run in Windows. Similarly video not showing up or running is a very common error. Smooth projection, all presentations opening up, all lettering seen without distortion or substitution, no blue screens, all videos running

Supplementary Information The online version contains supplementary material available at [https://doi.org/10.1007/978-981-19-1816-2_15].

A. J. Thakur, *Tapping the Power of PowerPoint for Medical Posters and Presentations*, https://doi.org/10.1007/978-981-19-1816-2_15

smoothly are coveted achievements for any conference organizing committee. Such a show does not just happen but needs to be organized meticulously.

Audiovisual Team

Audiovisual team (AV Team) is the most important unit of a conference organizing committee. It must be involved in planning from the very beginning and should be party to setting up objectives, conference design, and blueprint for the content. The AV Team should participate in the venue selection process. The number of attendees, number of simultaneous sessions, need for plenary and breakaway sessions, location of poster display, location of audiovisual booths, conference signage are important factors that decide the choice of a venue. There is an interdependence between a projected image and good visibility. The height of an image on the screen should be at least 20% of the length of the hall. If the hall is 100 feet long, then the screen should be 20 feet tall; only then the image will be well seen in the last row. The front row of the chairs should be at least 40 feet away for comfortable viewing. A 20 feet tall image is best visualized from chairs placed between 40 and 100 feet from the screen. The number of the expected audience dictates the size of the hall; the length of the hall dictates the size of the screen.

Importance of Audiovisual Features

Audiovisual aspect of a conference should be treated like a production of a film or drama. The individual presenters in a conference have the liberty to write their own script, but the presentations should follow good practices. These good practices should be defined by the AV Team for the conference and communicated to the prospective speakers. Left to themselves, each of the presenters will go by one's own conviction which may not be up to the standards desired by the 'director' of the show—the organizing committee. The Bombay Orthopaedic Society always sends out a document outlining the good presentation practices for their annual conference—WIROC® (Western India Regional Orthopaedic Conference). This document has had a positive effect on all the presenters irrespective of their standing in the speciality. There never is any regimentation or doctoring of an individual presentation, but mere suggestions to the speakers improve the quality of both, short and long presentations (Video 15.1).

Conference Schedule

The conference time table may be so arranged that various lecture sessions should start and end at staggered timings. There is strain on the infrastructure when all the rooms start and finish at the same time. Attendees are rushed from one hall to another, and often miss the beginning in the next session.

Hall Size and Aspect Ratio

The AV team should decide the screen's aspect ratio for a conference. Modern presentation programmes support outputs in two proportions. 4:3 and 16:9. A long and narrow hall, say 100 × 50 ft. should have presentations in 4:3 proportion. A long and wide hall, say 100 × 75 ft. should have presentations in 16:9 ratio. A uniform ratio in all the halls simplifies presentation handling in the preview room.

Types of Projection

The type of projection system for a conference should be settled in the beginning. Choice is between digital projection and LED walls. The images cast by electronic digital projector requires a certain degree of darkening of the hall for good visualization. In digital projection light backgrounds are suitable. Laser beam pointers are visible on the standard screens. LED walls are becoming popular, are expensive to rent, and require competent operators in the control booth. They display very radiant images that are visible in normal light. Standard laser pointers are ineffective on LED walls; a special pointing device is necessary to pinpoint an object on the screen. As the images seen on the LED walls are very bright, a presentation should be made with a dark background. The speakers should know the type of projection for their individual presentation so they can plan the background accordingly.

Emails for Communication

AV Team should have an independent email ID and should be communicated to all the speakers. Email exchanges should be attended by a senior member of the AV Team. The faculty likes prompt and definitive answers to their audiovisual needs; poor communication between the faculty and AV Team leads to audiovisual faux pas. The personnel for general management of a conference often fail to understand the nuances of AV arrangements and its importance to the faculty and for flawless conduct of the conference. Conference website should display FAQs, notes to the presenters and chairpersons.

Initial Audiovisual Planning

Final list of speakers at any conference matures gradually. The largest number of speakers make a presentation in the free papers segment. These are of short duration, 8–10 minutes including questions and answers. Most presenters in this group are younger members of the speciality. The AV Team should acquire their contact information like email and telephone numbers as soon as their submission is accepted for podium presentation. As more and more speakers accept invitations for longer formats, 25 and 50 minute talks, the same information should be collected from them. As and when the speakers' list is finalized the AV Team should write a 'note' to each of them individually giving a background of the audiovisual (AV) arrangements at the conference. The letter should mention the size of the audience, dimensions of the hall, and information that the presentation may be relayed to another hall where the presenter will not be visible. Other issues to be covered in the letter are: recommended version of PowerPoint or Keynote; aspect ratio (4:3, or 16:9) of the screen; type of computers to be used in lecture hall because presentations made in Keynote program will not run on Windows; type of projection system: digital projectors or LED walls; recommendation to use light background for digital projectors and dark background for LED walls; use of large fonts (at least 40 for the body and 46 for the title); to bring a copy of the software if a specialized font is used; quantity of text on a slide (one point per slide); advice to use all the available space to show a photo and not be bound by the programs' picture frames that reduce the size of the photo; suggestion to use animated block arrows and avoid use of laser pointer or computer mouse, to save time, increase accuracy, and be effective on multiple screens; advice to prepare slides with a view to use presenter view at the final delivery; instruction to coverup all the identifying text on investigative images and maintain patient's privacy; to use MP4 format for video; video to be inserted to run automatically; advice to ask for lavaliere mike for superior sound experience; plea to visit preview room at earliest, and submit the presentation after successful runs, particularly of videos. A hint in the cover letter that these are specific recommendations made by audiovisual experts for best image projection in this particular conference hall will secure cooperation of even the most vainglorious faculty. A copy of these recommendations should also be displayed on the conference website.

Second Communication

About 8 weeks before the conference each and every speaker should receive a detailed time table of the conference. Speakers always want to know what is happening around their presentation time. If there is a clash of interest, some of them may want to change the content of their presentation or seek other remedies. Not everyone stays for the entire conference. Once the final programme is published, the faculty can organize their travel arrangements. A 'reminder' copy of the 'note' to the speakers should also be sent along with this communication. Arrangements for remote submission of presentations should also be in place.

By this time, the list of chairpersons for each session should be ready. Each one should receive a copy of the final programme so they can organize one's time at the meeting. Chairperson is the organizing committee's representative for a particular session. Each one should receive a letter outlining the chair's role in the session (Fig. 15.1).

Expectations from a chairperson

- Be a 'tough, tougher, and toughest' chairperson
- Secure a copy of the conference programme and ensure conflict free time
- Acquire abstracts of the linked presentations; study them; formulate questions
- Learn pronunciations of the speakers' names
- Arrive early; know the functionaries in the hall
- Meet the speakers before the session
- Initiate the meeting as per schedule
- Irrespective of speaker's professional standing stop when time; be firm
- Question time: open it; regulate it; when time, end it
- Thank the speakers, thank the audience, and conclude the session

Fig. 15.1 Duties of a chairperson in a conference

The Preview Rooms

Preview room or speaker ready room is indispensable for smooth running of a large conference. It is the nerve centre of AV management. Its location should be easy to find. It is a place for all the speakers to check the presentation one last time and deposit it with the Preview room technical staff for timely display. The room should be spacious and have arrangements for faculty to sit down while waiting to load their presentations; they may utilize this time to chat with colleagues and old friends. Arrangements for snacks and beverages is a likeable adjunct to a preview room. Adequate number of technicians must be available in the preview room from an hour before the starting time and till the end of the day. It should have computers with the same software as one in use in the conference hall. Each and every presentation should be run in the preview room, correctly labelled for time, location, and speaker and then relayed to the designated hall. All the videos, irrespective of being embedded in or linked to the presentation, must be run in the preview room and glitches if present should be sorted out. All presentations are networked to the presentation rooms, therefore submission must be completed at least 30 minutes before the scheduled time.

Irrespective of the mode of submission, in person or remote uploading, a speaker must visit the preview room and run the presentation satisfactorily for at least a couple of times to ensure flawless performance. This is imperative if the presentation has videos and animations. Videos make or break a conference. These are fun to watch provided they work well on cue. However, videos universally follow Murphy's Law: if anything is likely to go wrong, it will. To beat Murphy at his game the videos should be converted to one of the following types: AVI/WMV/MP4 format. There are hundreds of video formats; each camera company has one for each of its models and so on. The three formats mentioned above are simplest and work well universally on all the machines. Conversion is easy; most computers have a converter program or one may download free software from website https://handbrake.fr/ or purchase from https://compressor.io/ or https://www.videoproc.com/. 'Run automatic' option should be chosen when inserting a video in the presentation. Should the video start before its time, it may be controllable with a click of a button. With the option to 'start on click', the computer often wastes several moments before the images move, squanders the presenter's precious time and the audience loses patience.

Lavaliere mike and Presenter View

The faculty gets an opportunity in the preview room to make minor corrections like fonts which may show differently than intended. Special needs, like lavaliere mike, presenter view, step-up platform for short persons, etc., should be notified to the technicians. Lavaliere mics are best for large conferences because they carry the speaker's voice efficiently (Fig. 15.2a). Speaker has the ease of moving around and

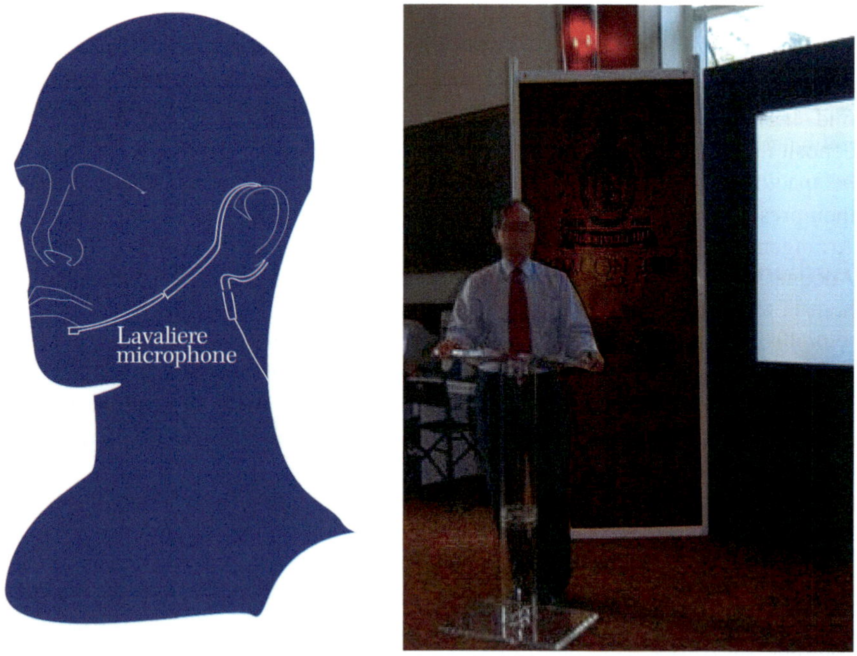

A B

Fig. 15.2 (**a**) Lavaliere mike (**b**) replica lectern with buttons similar to one in the lecture hall. The stage like setup offers photo-opportunity looking in any direction without the fear of dropping his audibility. Fixed-mike on a lectern is a standard provision in a conference. It needs practice to use this device effectively. One has to be close to the mike all the time; any movement away from it causes a drop in the clarity; most medical speakers use this apparatus poorly. Speakers should always insist on Lavaliere mike for superior voice delivery. Use of the presenter's view is advantageous. It helps the speaker to reduce the number of text slides as he can 'read' his text covertly, see the next slide before the audience to his advantage, and effectively control the progress of the presentation. However, the AV Team must let the speakers know in advance the availability of presenter view, so they can modify their presentation to take full advantage of the facility.

Replica Lectern

In the preview room display of a mock lectern with accurate reproduction of the features in use in the lecture hall helps the presenters to get acquainted with the function of the buttons and other finer artefacts of the lectern; each one of the speakers may not be able to check the arrangements in the actual hall. Using a model lectern helps some speakers to get over the nerves and they may practice here for the final time under simulated conditions. It also serves as a setup for a commemorative photograph for novice speakers (Fig. 15.2b). Laser pointers are often available on the lectern but the screens are large and one may waste several precious seconds to spot the point of interest. Besides, a laser pointer is ineffective as multiple screens are used for judges and chairpersons; additionally laser pointers are ineffective when LED walls are used for display. The presenters should use computer generated animated arrows; with a click of a button an arrow appears at the precise point and serves the purpose.

Audience Response Systems

Audience response systems (ARS) also known as personal response system, or electronic voting system, helps the audience to answer displayed multiple choice questions using a remote control device. All responses are collated and instantly presented, in chart forms—a bar graph, a pie chart, or a line graph, and projected on a screen in real time. This is a great device for getting feedback. In the present time, smart phones can be used for responses and there is no need for a separate handheld device. It is not necessary for all the respondents to be in one location. It can also be used over the Internet, thus making it useful in a webinar.

The system depends on the ability of the faculty to write multiple choice questions on topics under discussion. This adds to preparation time, needs practice and training. Initial warm up question induces the attendees to focus on the material being presented. People then pay attention and remain engaged because they are expected to answer; this improves learning percentages. ARS promotes active interaction and discussion among the attendees and the faculty. It is useful in explaining and clarifying concepts; asking questions clears many doubts. Since answers are anonymous all attendees participate without reservation. The ARS improves the quality of meetings by making them more engaging, inclusive, and productive. It is especially useful in CMEs and in meetings that are designed to promote discussion between attendees and faculty.

Hall Arrangements

In a lecture hall, the light switch should be close to the technician's booth to dim the lights as and when required. A technician should be close at hand at the lectern, as technical help may be required during the proceedings. Nearer the technician's desk to the lectern, the better the coordination with the presenter. However, this arrangement is dictated by local layout. Organizers often appoint one middle level person as room controller who oversees the ongoing events. Multiple stand-alone mikes are placed in the auditorium to enable the audience to ask questions. The mikes should be numbered; it helps the chair to control the Q & A session.

Sponsored Sessions

Certain sessions are sponsored by commercial entities. This may include selection of the topics and the speakers by the sponsor. When such an arrangement exists, the conference committee should make a clear statement to that effect. This is an ethical requirement. The audience should know why they are listening to a speaker on a particular topic.

Magical meetings emanate from audiovisual committee's astute planning and hard work.

Index

A. J. Thakur, *Tapping the Power of PowerPoint for Medical Posters and Presentations*, https://doi.org/10.1007/978-981-19-1816-2

GPSR Compliance

The European Union's (EU) General Product Safety Regulation (GPSR) is a set of rules that requires consumer products to be safe and our obligations to ensure this.

If you have any concerns about our products, you can contact us on ProductSafety@springernature.com

In case Publisher is established outside the EU, the EU authorized representative is:

Springer Nature Customer Service Center GmbH
Europaplatz 3
69115 Heidelberg, Germany

Batch number: 10726135

Printed by Printforce, the Netherlands